W0050498

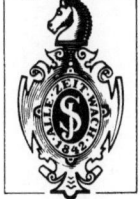

T. H. Moss

Tumours of the Nervous System

an Ultrastructural Atlas

With 120 Figures

Springer-Verlag
London Berlin Heidelberg New York
Paris Tokyo

T. H. Moss, MB, ChB, PhD, MRCPath
Department of Neuropathology
Frenchay Hospital
Bristol BS16 1LE

ISBN-13: 978-1-4471-1428-4   e-ISBN-13: 978-1-4471-1426-0
DOI:10.1007/ 978-1-4471-1426-0

The work is subject to copyright. All rights are reserved, whether the whole or part of the material is concerned, specifically those of translation, reprinting, re-use of illustrations, broadcasting, reproduction by photocopying machine or similar means, and storage in data banks. Under §54 of the German Copyright Law where copies are made for other than private use, a fee is payable to 'Verwertungsgesellschaft Wort', Munich.

© Springer-Verlag Berlin Heidelberg 1986
Softcover reprint of the hardcover 1st edition 1986

The use of registered names, trademarks, etc. in this publication does not imply, even in the absence of a specific statement, that such names are exempt from the relevant protective laws and regulations and therefore free for general use.

Product Liability : The publisher can give no guarantee for information about drug dosage and application thereof contained in this book. In every individual case the respective user must check its accuracy by consulting other pharmaceutical literature.

2128/3916 543210

Preface

Since the time of the earliest electron microscopic studies on tumours of the human nervous system, undertaken over 20 years ago by Luse and her colleagues, there have been considerable advances in our understanding of these neoplasms. Tissue culture and specific antibodies to tumour antigens are two of the techniques which have greatly aided such advances, enabling much to be learned about the biological properties and underlying nature of all types of nervous system tumour. Electron microscopy, however, has continued to prove of considerable value in the investigation of these tumours, and the technological advances of the last two decades have dramatically improved the resolution and overall quality of the ultrastructural images obtained. In clinical neuropathology, such improvements have encouraged a more widespread use of the electron microscope in the diagnosis of human nervous system tumours, alongside antibody techniques and more conventional histological methods. Although ultrastructural examination is often not strictly necessary to identify well-differentiated tumours such as astrocytomas or choroid plexus papillomas, study of the electron microscopic features in such cases frequently proves useful in the diagnosis of their more malignant counterparts. Thus the recognition of astrocytic filaments in anaplastic gliomas, or of cilia in pleomorphic choroid plexus carcinomas, may enable a diagnosis to be made in cases where there is insufficient differentiation for the tumours to be recognised at light microscopic level.

This atlas has been designed principally as a diagnostic aid for clinical neuropathologists, although some features of academic interest have also been included, especially where the true nature and cellular origins of a tumour are still uncertain. In each group of tumours,well-differentiated examples have been chosen for illustration, in the hope that familiarity with the typical features of a given type of tumour will help in the diagnosis of the more difficult cases with less characteristic appearances. The list of tumours included is by no means exhaustive, but most of the types commonly encountered in routine neuropathological practice are represented, together with some of the more important rare forms, such as pineoblastoma and ganglioglioma. The space devoted to the various types of tumour is not proportional to the frequency of their occurrence, but reflects the number and variety of specific ultrastructural features which may be found, and thus the diagnostic potential of electron microscopy in each case. As a result, tumours such as astrocytomas have been given rather sparse attention relative to their importance in clinical practice, whereas tumours like neuroblastomas, which can often pose a diagnostic problem, have been extensively illustrated despite their relative rarity. In some other cases, tumours which are usually easily diagnosed without the help of electron microscopy have been closely scrutinised because of current interest in their pathogenesis or differentiating capacity, as for example with subependymomas and medulloblastomas.

Finally, it is worth emphasising that the effectiveness of electron microscopy as a diagnostic technique is at least partly dependent on the way the tissue is handled, and factors such as delay prior to fixation may seriously impair the ability to recognise important ultrastructural features. For this reason, all the illustrations in this atlas were made from glutaraldehyde-fixed neurosurgical biopsy material, and although some variation in the quality of tissue preservation has been unavoidable, no pictures of formalin-fixed or post-mortem material have been included.

Bristol, England, 1986   T. H. Moss

Acknowledgements

The quality of these electron micrographs is a considerable tribute to the expert and patient technical assistance of Mr. T. Gradidge, who was responsible both for the preparation of the ultrathin sections and for the printing of the photographic plates. The wide variety of glutaraldehyde-fixed biopsy material on which this atlas is based was collected over several years in the Department of Neuropathology, Frenchay Hospital, Bristol, by Dr. D. B. Brownell, who has also provided invaluable encouragement and advice during the completion of the project. Any ultrastructural study of tumour biopsies depends implicitly on the care taken by the surgeon to provide suitable tissue at the time of operation, and for this the author gratefully acknowledges the untiring cooperation and enthusiasm of the Frenchay Hospital neurosurgeons, Mr. H. B. Griffith, Mr. B. H. Cummins, Mr. M. J. Torrens and Mr. H. B. Coakham. Finally, but by no means of least importance, thanks are due to Mrs. P. Penfold, who typed all the manuscripts with great dedication.

Contents

1 Astrocytoma

The fibrillary and protoplasmic forms of astrocytoma are not clearly defined at ultrastructural level, and the majority of tumours show a spectrum of intermediate appearances. Both fibrillary and protoplasmic tumour cells are present in all cases, but in variable proportions, with one or other cell type predominating in many examples.

In the more protoplasmic type of tumour, the predominant cell resembles a non-neoplastic protoplasmic astrocyte and has prominent, often bipolar cell processes. These contain both 20-nm microtubules and 6- to 9-nm glial filaments, and may be joined to each other by zonulae adherentes junctions. The nuclei are typically irregular or lobulated in shape and have marginated chromatin. Glial filaments are scarce or entirely absent in the perikaryal cytoplasm, but other organelles are usually abundant and include membrane-bound vesicles and rough endoplasmic reticulum. In microcystic tumours, the cystic spaces are visible ultrastructurally as separate, rounded loculi of extracellular space enclosed by basement membrane. Although not associated with blood vessels, these basement membrane microcysts have tumour cell foot processes attached to their outer surfaces, similar to those present around vascular basement membranes.

The cell predominating in more fibrillary astrocytomas resembles a non-neoplastic fibrillary astrocyte, and differs from the protoplasmic cell type in having abundant 6- to 9-nm glial filaments in the perikaryal cytoplasm as well as in the cell processes. Other cytoplasmic organelles are often rather sparse and tend to be displaced by the perikaryal filaments, which are often perinuclear in distribution. Electron-dense Rosenthal bodies may occur in close association with the glial filaments in fibrillary cell types, and possibly represent the result of increased production or diminished degradation of filament protein. The ultrastructural equivalent of a carrot-shaped Rosenthal fibre is a tumour cell process distended by a large mass of similar electron-dense material.

In gemistocytic astrocytomas, most of the cells have flattened, eccentric nuclei and massively enlarged cytoplasm, which shows little tendency to form peripheral processes. The voluminous cytoplasm may contain a variety of diffusely scattered organelles, but is mostly filled by a meshwork of haphazardly orientated, short lengths of 6- to 9-nm glial filaments.

The most prominent architectural feature of all types of astrocytoma at ultrastructural level is the greatly expanded extracellular space, in which the tumour cell processes form a tenuous, complex and loose meshwork. Blood vessels have an essentially normal structure and tumour cells form astrocytic-type foot processes around their outer basement membranes. In contrast to normal central nervous tissue, however, the foot process layer is often incomplete in astrocytomas, and this feature has been associated with the breakdown in blood–brain barrier known to occur in these tumours.

Further Reading

Duffel D, Farber L, Chou S, Hartmann JB, Nelson E (1963) Electron microscopic observations on astrocytomas. Subependymal glomerulate astrocytoma. Am J Pathol 43: 539–545

Ebhardt G, Cervós-Navarro J (1981) The fine structure of cells in astrocytomas of various grades of malignancy. Acta Neuropathol 7: 88–90

Hossmann KA, Wechsler W (1971) Ultrastructural cytopathology of human cerebral gliomas. Oncology 25: 455–480

Luse SA (1960) Electron microscopic studies of brain tumours. Neurology 10: 881–905

Zülch KJ, Wechsler W (1968) Pathology and classification of gliomas. In: Krayenbuhl H, Maspes PE, Sweet WH (eds) Progress in neurological surgery, vol 2. Karger, Basel, pp 1–84

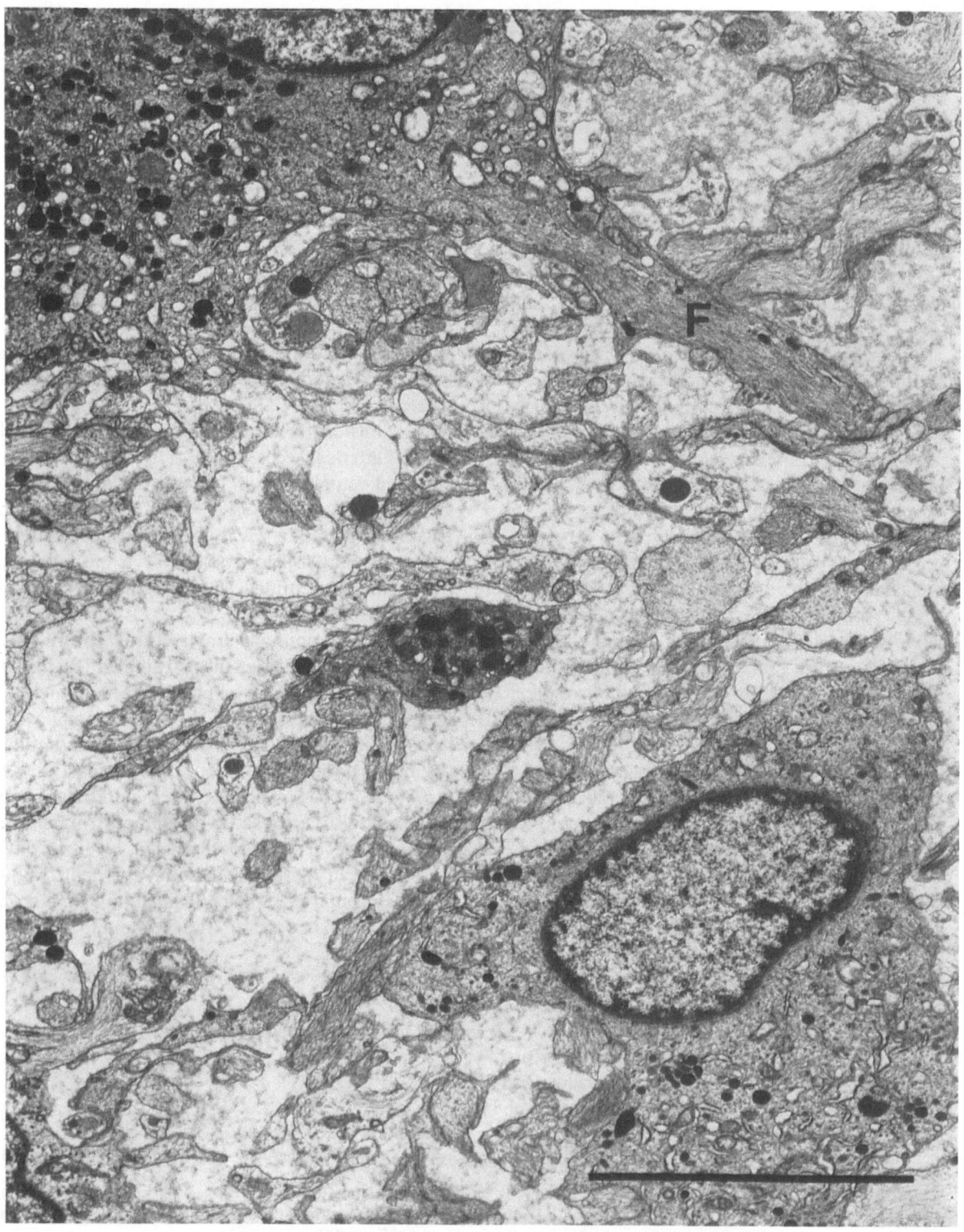

Fig. 1.1. *Protoplasmic astrocytoma.* The cells predominating in these tumours show similarities with non-neoplastic, protoplasmic astrocytes. Like the cells seen here, they usually have abundant and varied organelles in the perikaryal cytoplasm, but glial filaments are scanty or absent in this region. By contrast, the irregular peripheral processes are filled with 6- to 9-nm glial filaments (*F*), and form a loose meshwork in the greatly expanded extracellular space. (Bar = 5 μm)

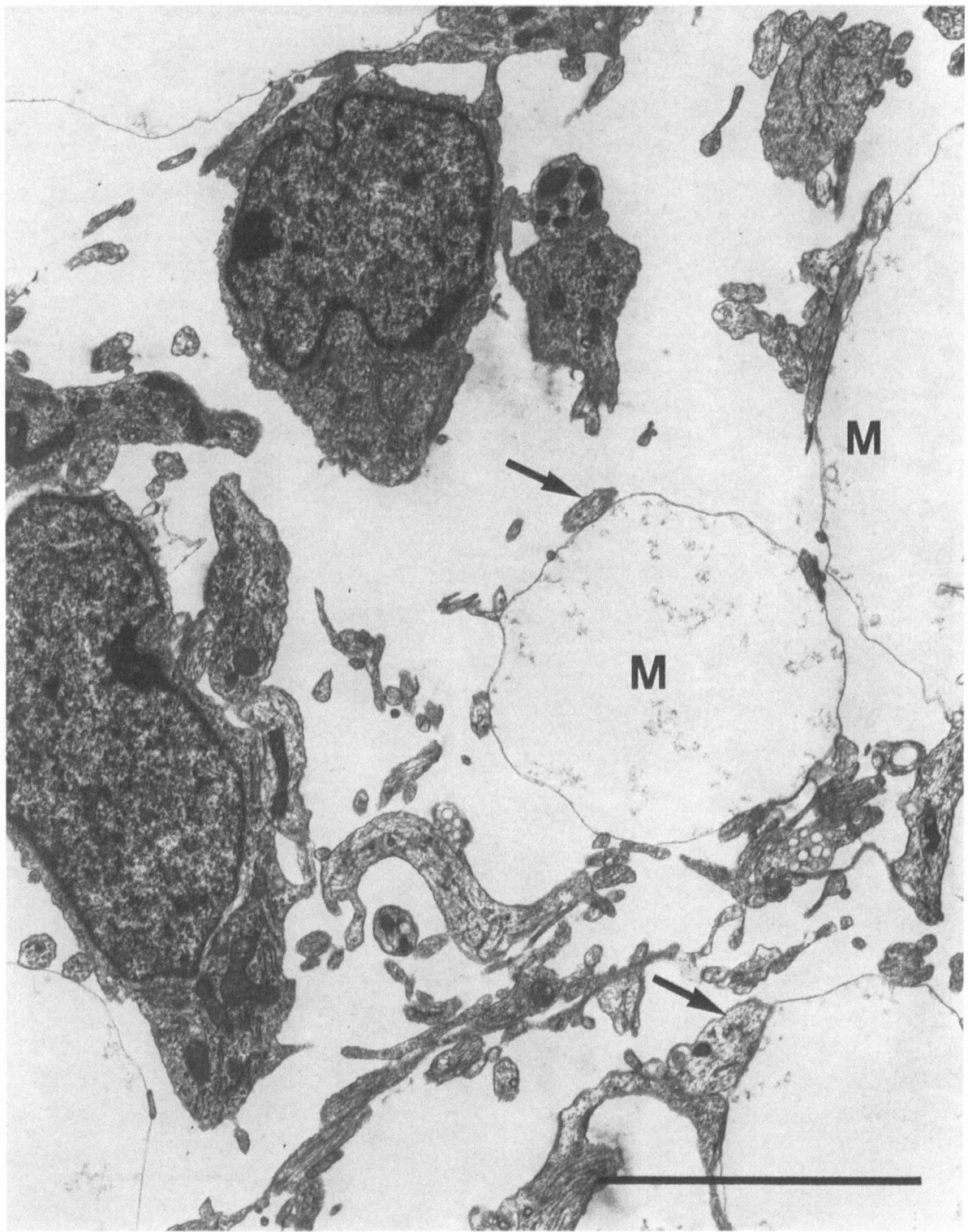

Fig. 1.2. *Microcystic protoplasmic astrocytoma.* The microcystic spaces (*M*) are enclosed by basement membrane, and attached to their outer surfaces they have tumour cell foot processes (*arrows*) similar to those found around vascular basement membranes. The tumour cells shown here are of protoplasmic type and lack perikaryal filaments. The expanded extracellular space seen in this figure is a characteristic feature of all types of low-grade astrocytoma. (Bar = 5 μm)

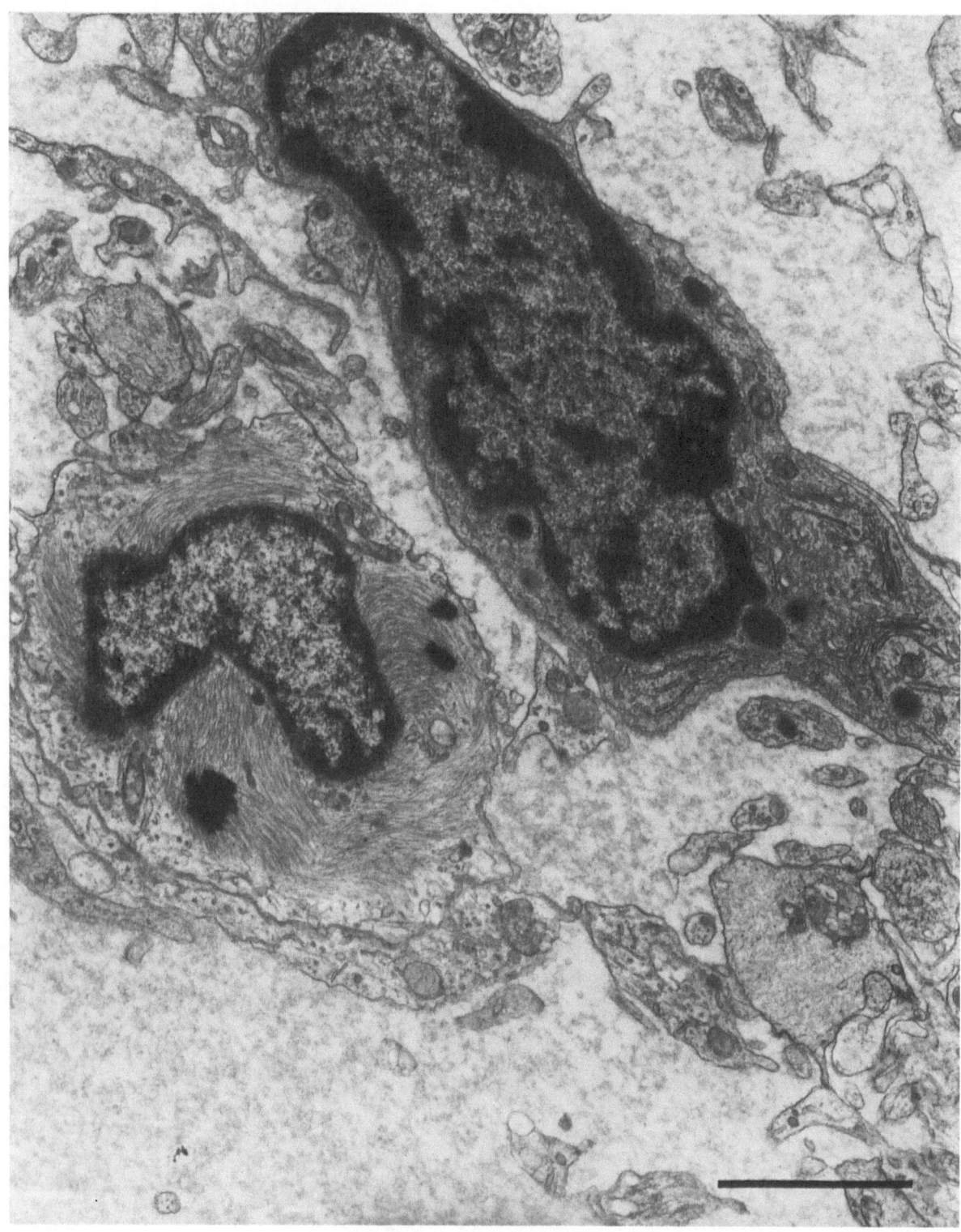

Fig. 1.3. *Fibrillary astrocytoma.* The predominant cells in these tumours resemble non-neoplastic fibrillary astrocytes and, like the cell seen on the *left*, usually have abundant 6- to 9-nm glial filaments in their perikaryal cytoplasm. These filaments may be closely associated with electron-dense condensations, or Rosenthal bodies, as in this example. Protoplasmic cell types, like that on the *right*, may also be present in these tumours and lack perikaryal filaments. In both cell types the nuclei are usually irregular in shape with marginated chromatin. (Bar = 2 μm)

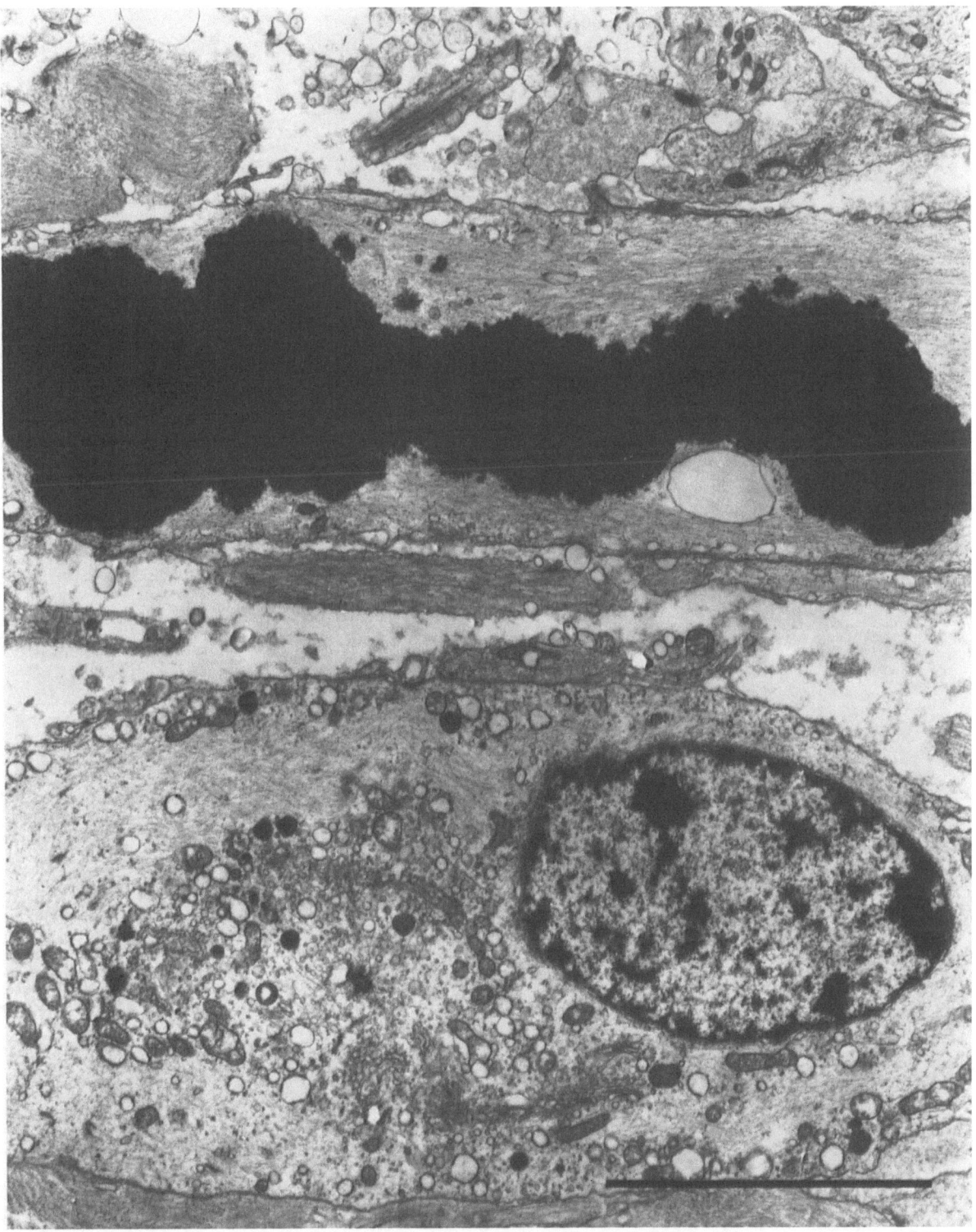

Fig. 1.4. *Pilocytic fibrillary astrocytoma.* These tumours are formed almost entirely of fibrillary-type cells with abundant perikaryal filaments, like the cell in the *lower part* of this figure. Rosenthal fibres, like the one seen above this cell, consist ultrastructurally of an irregular mass of electron-dense material in a swollen, filament-containing tumour cell process. (Bar = 5 μm)

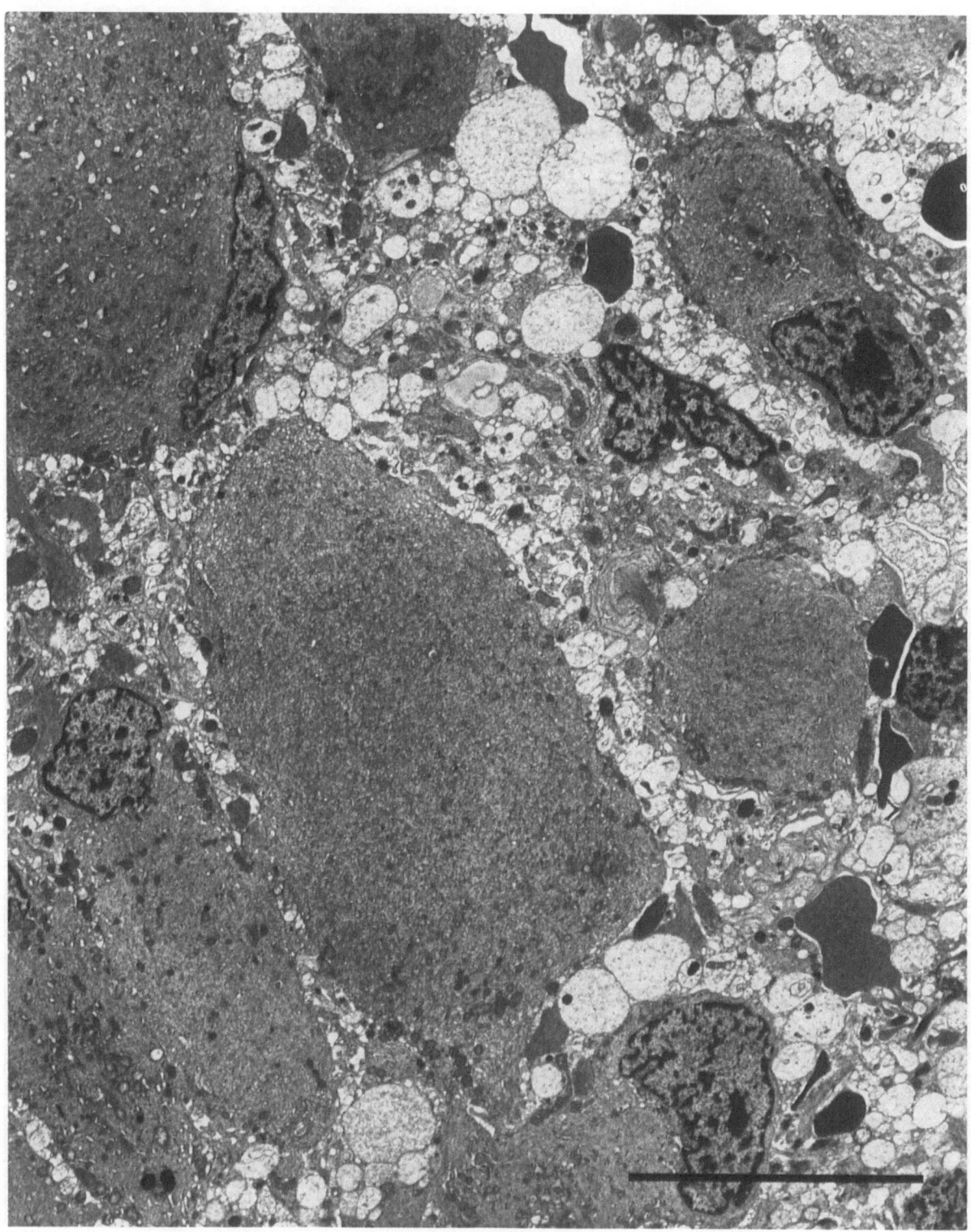

Fig. 1.5. *Gemistocytic astrocytoma.* The grossly enlarged cells of these tumours have a characteristic appearance, with eccentric nuclei, voluminous cytoplasm and little tendency to form peripheral processes. Those seen in this figure are infiltrating non-neoplastic neuropil. (Bar = 10 μm)

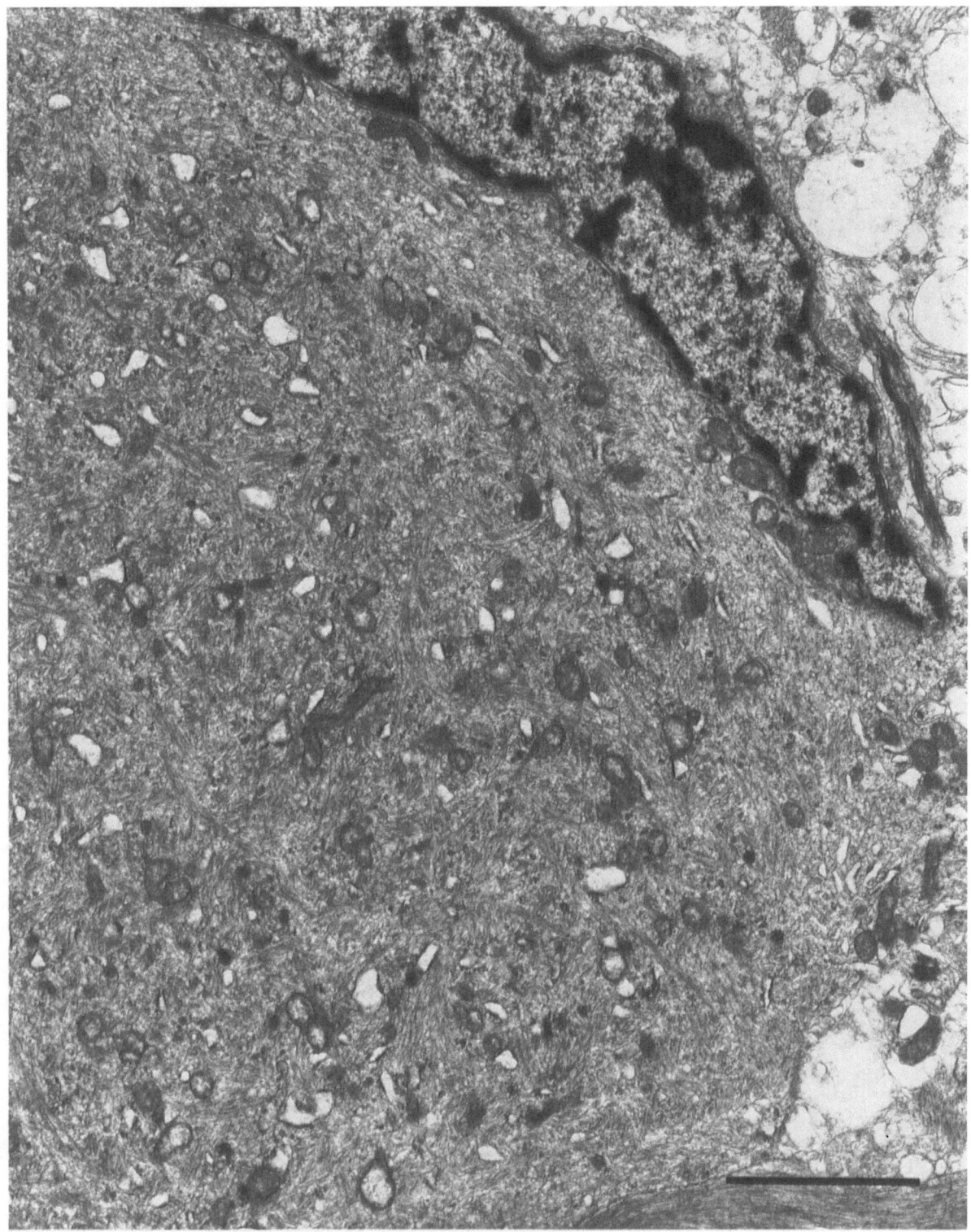

Fig. 1.6. *Gemistocytic astrocytoma.* The tumour cells contain diffusely scattered organelles of varying type, but as can be seen here, the voluminous cytoplasm is largely filled by a meshwork of randomly arranged, short lengths of 6- to 9-nm glial filaments. (Bar = 2 μm)

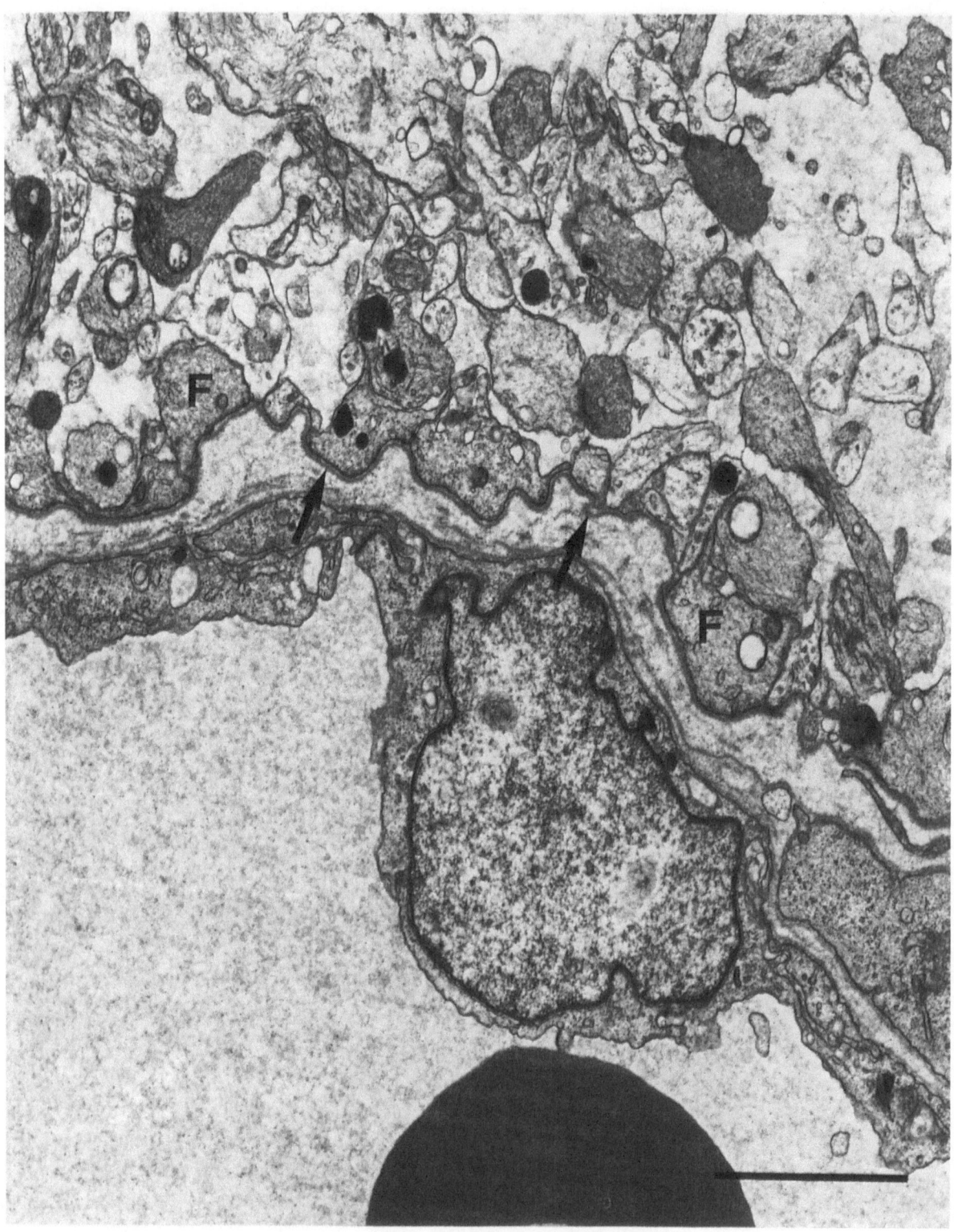

Fig. 1.7. *Fibrillary astrocytoma.* The capillaries in all types of astrocytoma have an essentially normal structure, with a layer of tumour cell foot processes (*F*) around the outer (glial) basement membrane (*arrows*). Although apparently complete in the area shown here, this neoplastic foot process layer may be patchy in some places. (Bar = 2 μm)

2 Oligodendroglioma

Away from their infiltrating margins, oligodendrogliomas form relatively solid sheets of cells with little intervening extracellular space. Many of the cells show similarities to normal oligodendroglia, with abundant, electron-lucent perikaryal cytoplasm and regular, rounded nuclei. Nuclear chromatin is typically finely granular and there may be a prominent nucleolus. The cytoplasm contains only scanty ribosomes and endoplasmic reticulum, but mitochondria are often abundant and may fill the entire cell. In some cases, the mitochondria may be abnormally large or have a deranged architecture, and those with an elongated, skein-like appearance have been called "fusiform membranous bodies". Although adjacent cell membranes are often closely apposed, junctional attachments are either entirely absent or represented only by small, punctate membrane densities. The tumour cell bodies are frequently separated by sheets of electron-lucent, interdigitating processes containing 20-nm microtubules. These cell processes show a marked tendency towards a lamellar organisation, with parallel bundles of thin processes arranged crescentically or concentrically around cell bodies. They may also form tighter, more discrete spirals known as "concentric membrane structures", which are thought to represent an attempt at primitive myelin sheath formation. A second, smaller cell type may also be present, with scanty and more electron-dense cytoplasm containing few organelles. A similar variation of cytoplasmic electron density also occurs in normal oligodendroglia, and may represent the state of cell hydration at the time of fixation. In oligodendroglioma, however, it has also been suggested that the small, darker cells are more primitive, and may eventually mature into the larger, pale ones. Typical, filament-containing astrocytic cells are often dispersed throughout the tumour, but in addition some of the oligodendroglial-like tumour cells may also contain 6- to 9-nm glial filaments, or even Rosenthal bodies. These cells possibly represent an embryonal form of astrocyte, but have also been interpreted as evidence of astrocytic differentiation in oligodendroglial tumour cells. Blood vessel architecture is essentially normal, but tumour cell processes usually envelop the intact outer, glial, basement membrane in a randomly orientated fashion, without a regular layer of foot processes.

Further Reading

Cervós-Navarro J (1981) Ultrastructure of oligodendrogliomas. Acta Neuropathol [Suppl] 7: 91–93

Garcia JH, Lemini H (1970) Ultrastructure of oligodendroglioma of the spinal cord. Am J Clin Pathol 54: 757–765

Hossmann KA, Wechsler W (1971) Ultrastructural cytopathology of human cerebral gliomas. Oncology 25: 455–480

Luse A (1960) Electron microscopic studies of brain tumours. Neurology 10: 881–905

Robertson DM, Vogel FS (1962) Concentric lamination of glial processes in oligodendrogliomas. J Cell Biol 15: 313–334

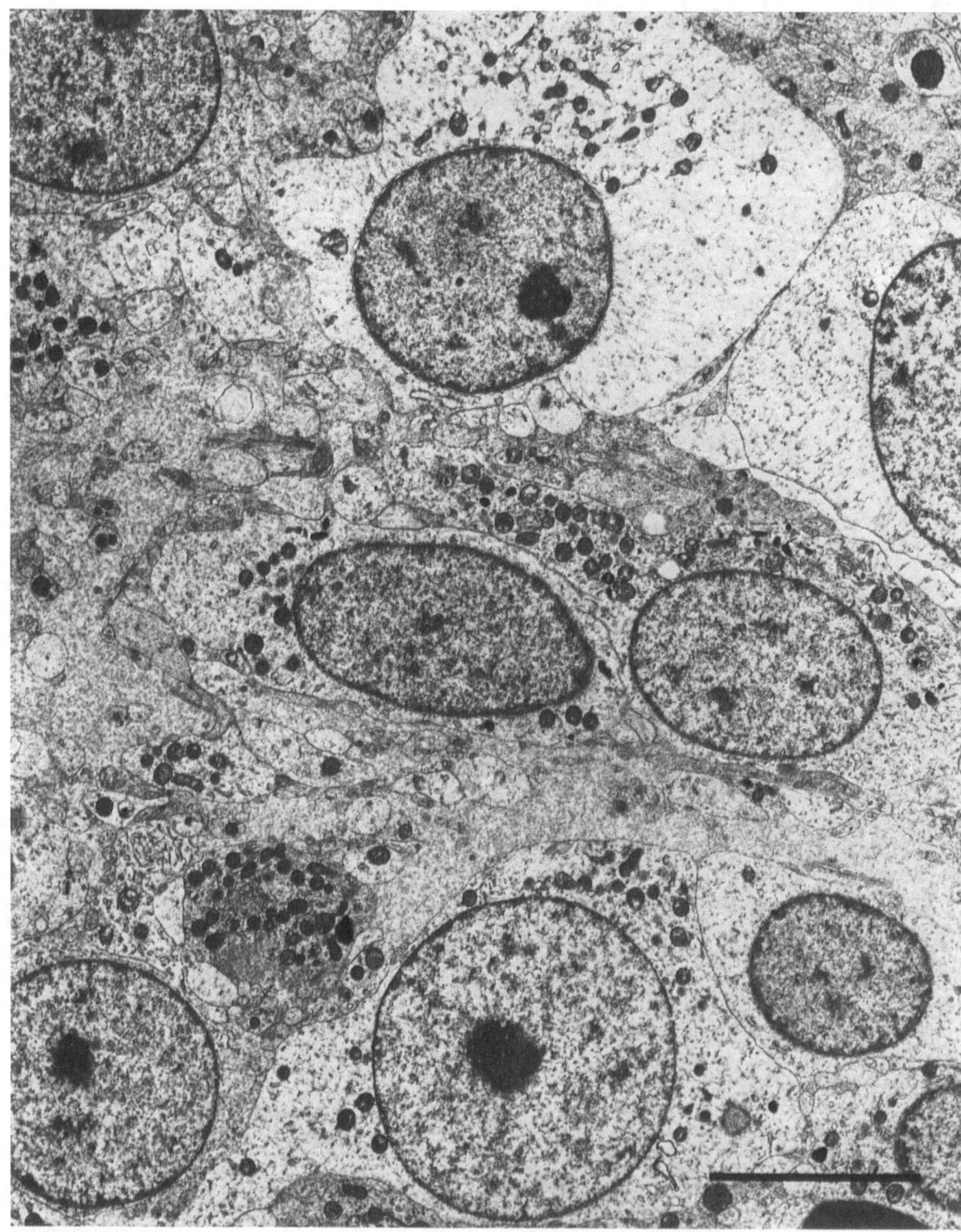

Fig. 2.1. *Oligodendroglioma.* The tumour cells tend to be arranged in monotonous sheets and often show similarities with non-neoplastic oligodendroglia. Like the cells shown here, they usually have uniform, round nuclei with prominent nucleoli. The abundant, electron-lucent perinuclear cytoplasm typically has an empty appearance and contains rather scanty organelles. Some of the cell bodies may be separated by pale-staining processes, like those seen around the cells in the *centre*. (Bar = 5 μm)

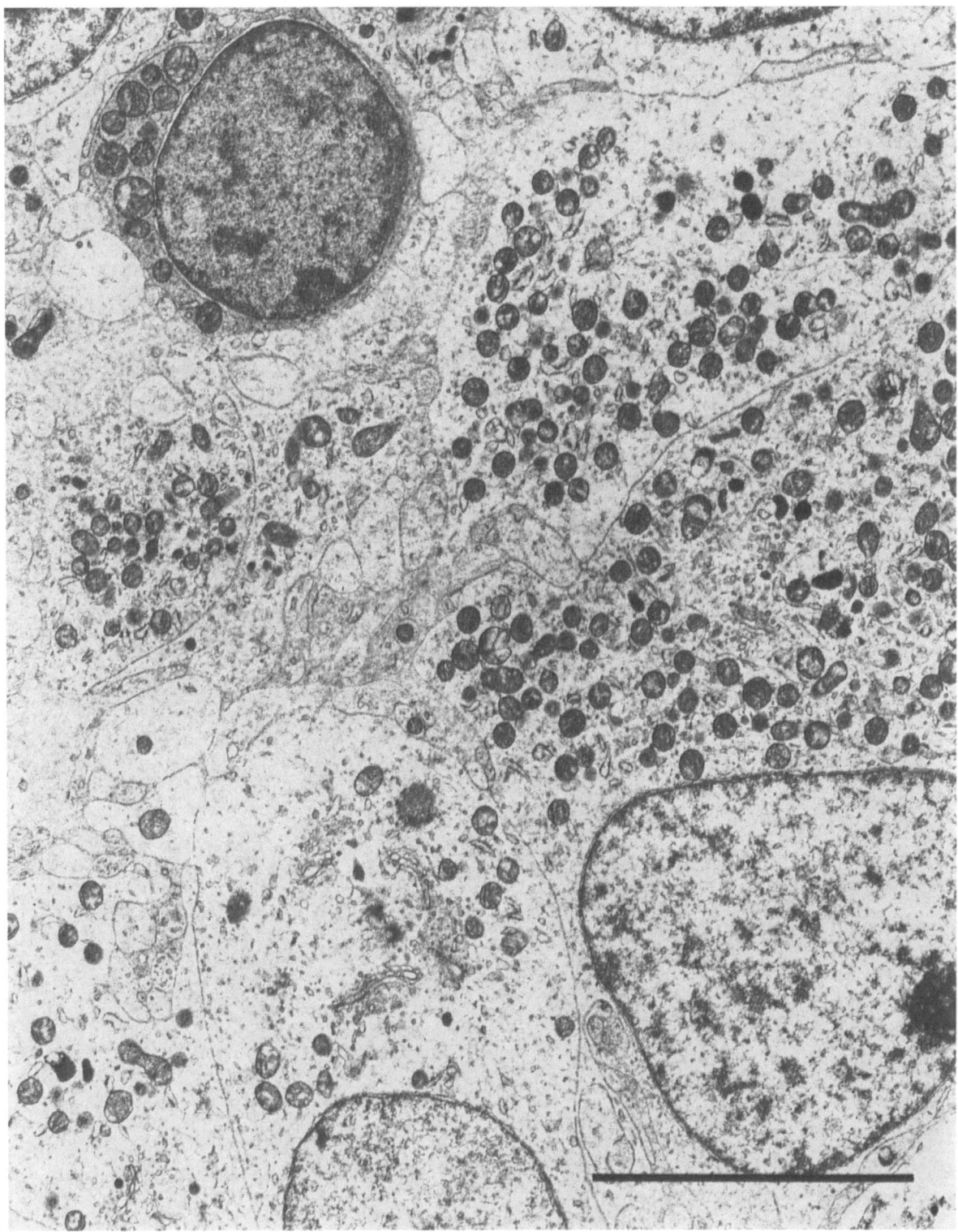

Fig. 2.2. *Oligodendroglioma.* Cytoplasmic organelles are generally rather sparse, but some cells may contain abundant mitochondria, as in the examples shown here. The cell bodies are generally tightly apposed but do not form junctional attachments. A second, smaller type of tumour cell may also be present, like the one seen at the *top,* and has scanty, more electron-dense cytoplasm. (Bar = 5 μm)

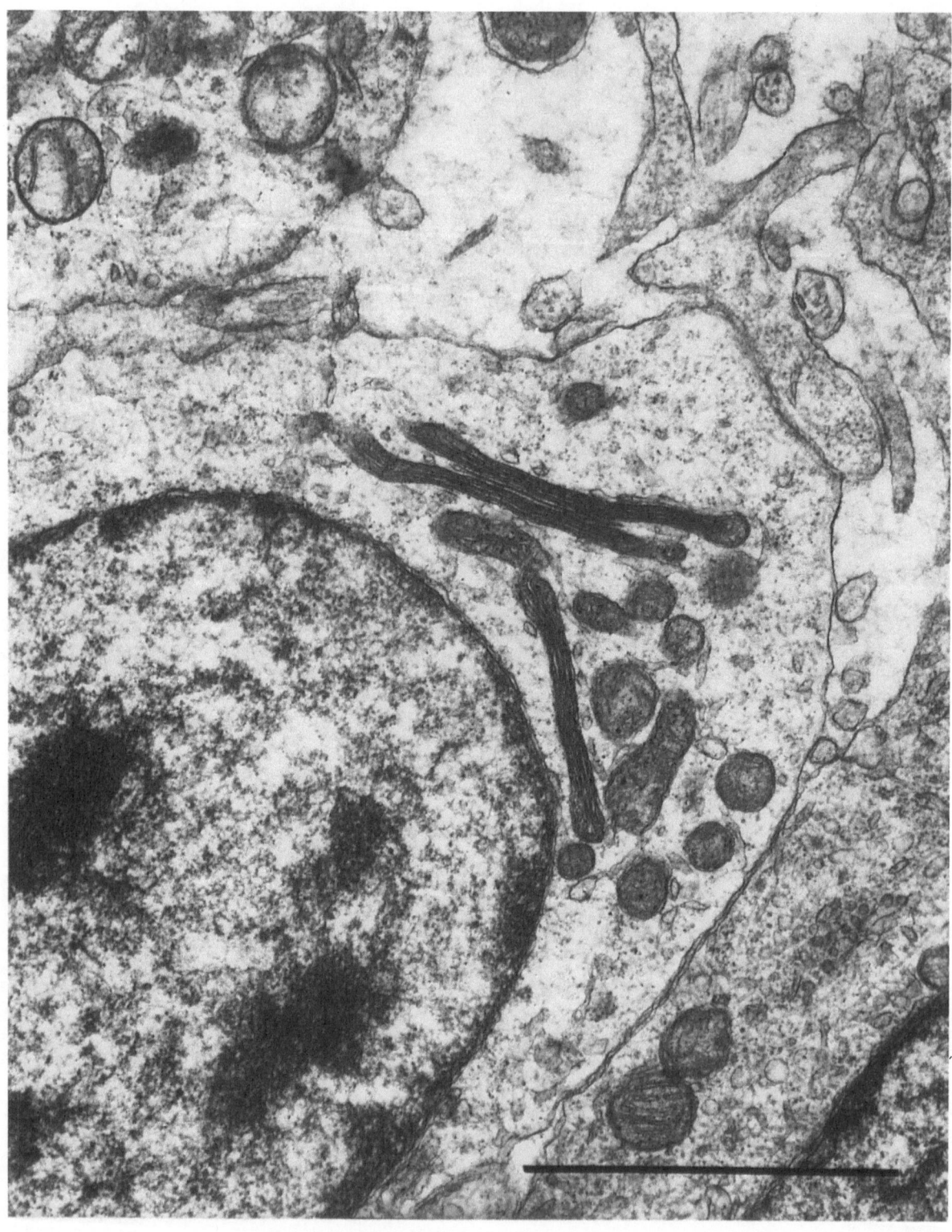

Fig. 2.3. *Oligodendroglioma.* In some tumour cells, mitochondria may be unusually large or have a deranged architecture. The abnormally elongated, skein-like mitochondria seen in this cell have been called "fusiform membranous bodies". (Bar = 2 μm)

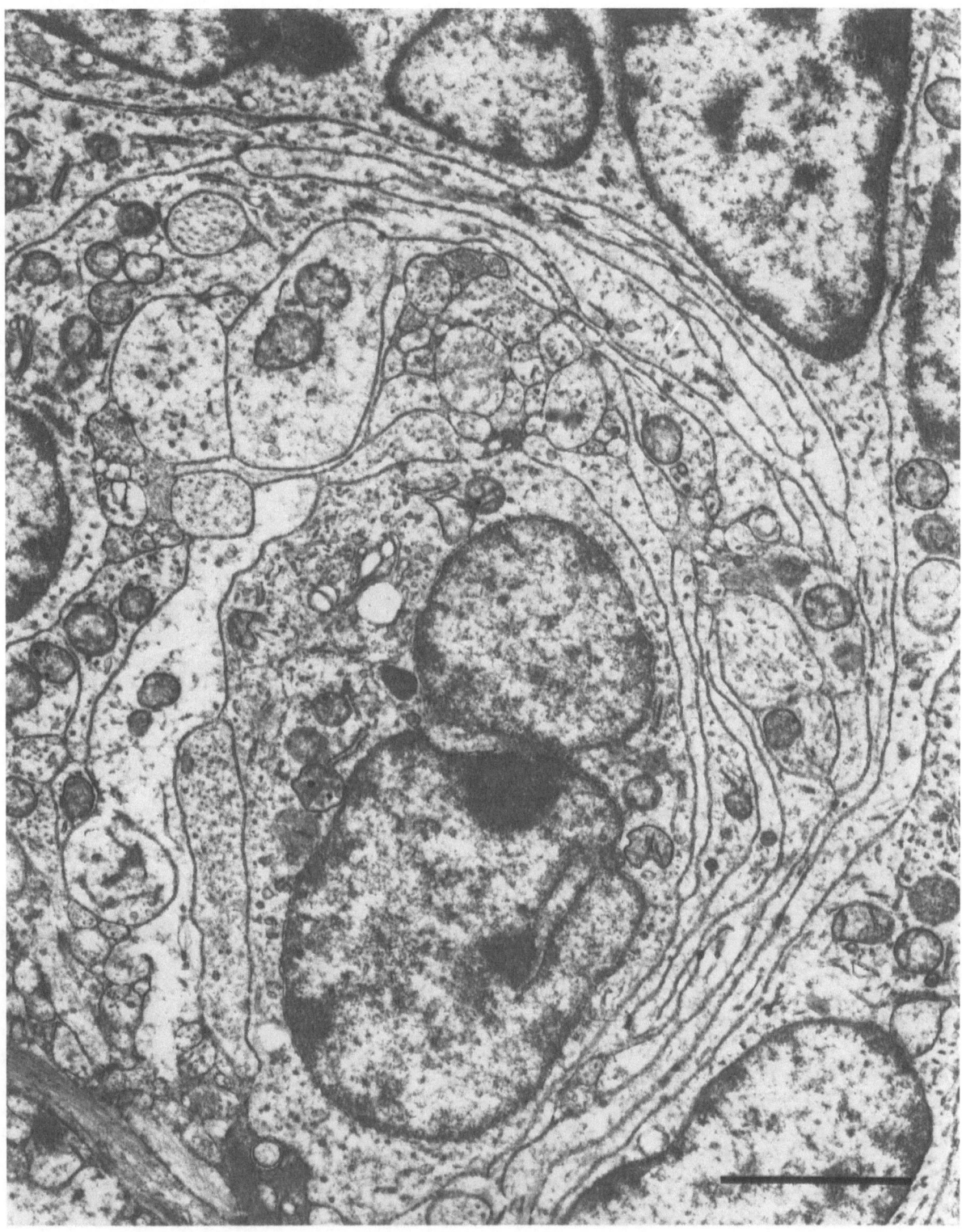

Fig. 2.4. *Oligodendroglioma.* The electron-lucent tumour cell processes are typically arranged in parallel bundles and may show a crescentic or lamellar organisation around central cell bodies, as in this field. (Bar = 2 μm)

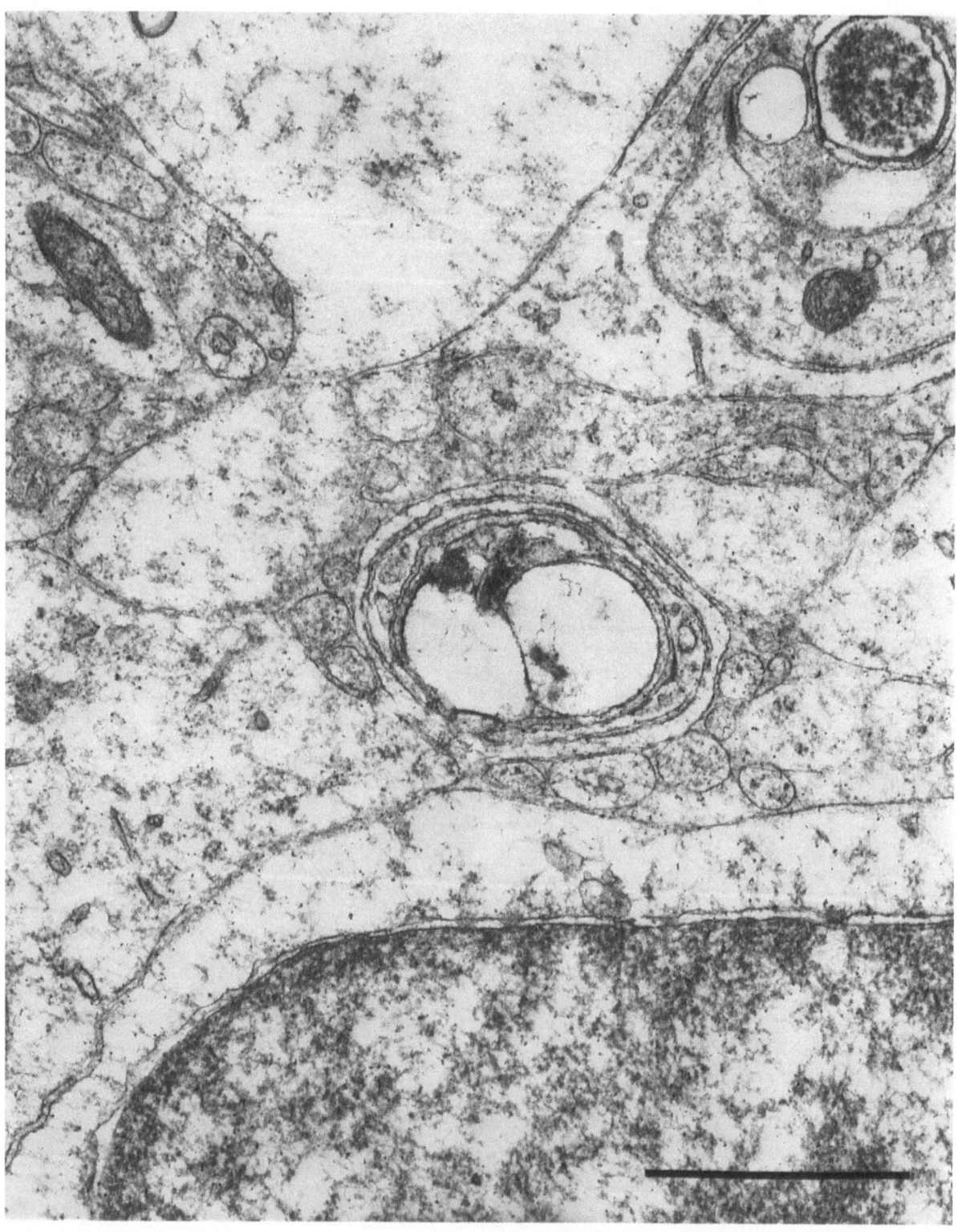

Fig. 2.5. *Oligodendroglioma.* Attenuated tumour cell processes may occasionally form discrete, tight spirals, like the one shown here. These spirals are sometimes referred to as "concentric membrane structures", and are thought to represent a primitive attempt at myelin sheath formation. (Bar = 1 µm)

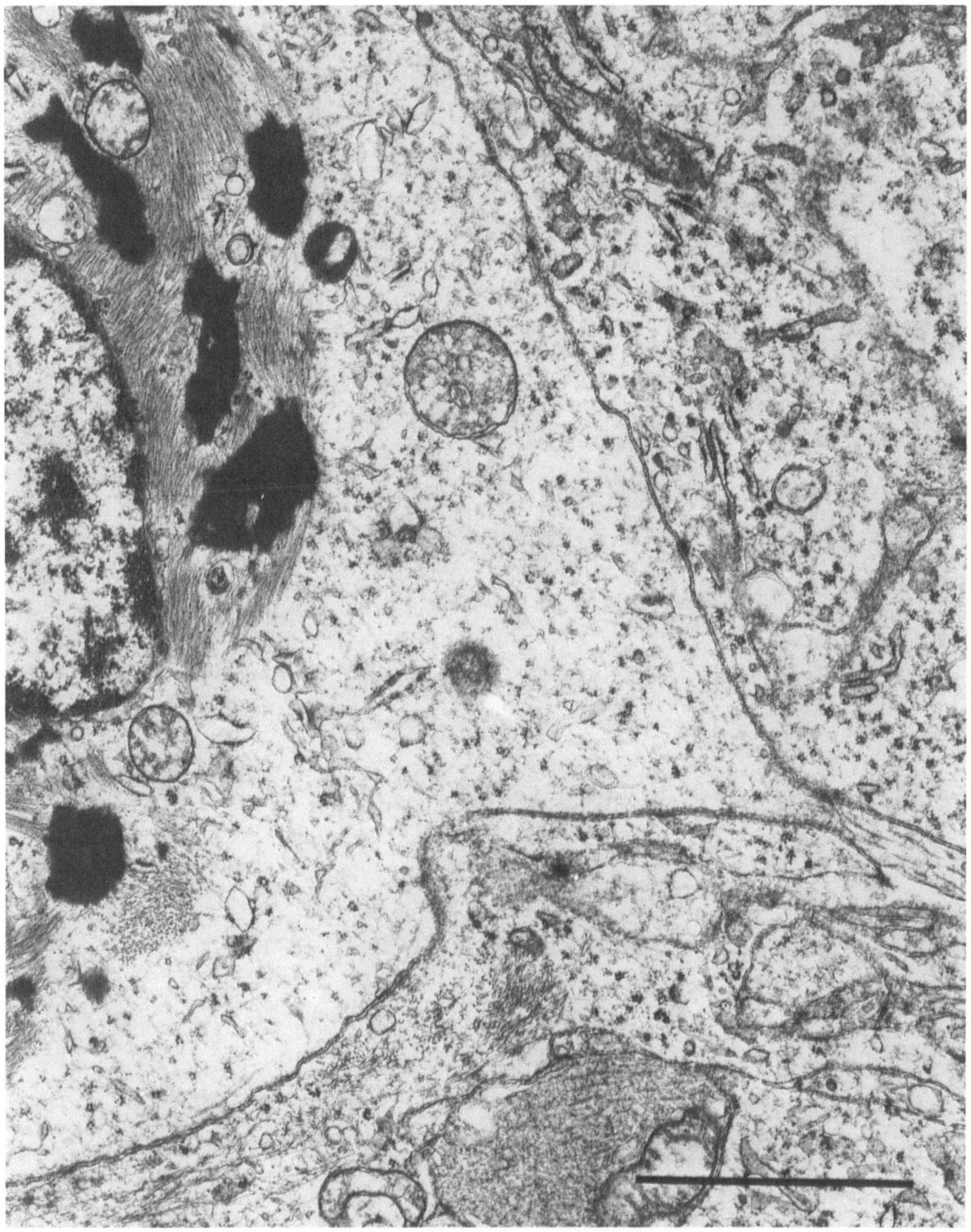

Fig. 2.6. *Oligodendroglioma.* Some otherwise typical, oligodendroglial-like tumour cells may have bundles of 6- to 9-nm glial filaments in their perikaryal cytoplasm. These filaments are occasionally associated with electron-dense Rosenthal bodies, as in this example. Such cells have been interpreted as evidence of true astrocytic differentiation in neoplastic oligodendroglial cells, and have been dubbed "gliofibrillary oligodendrocytes". (Bar = 2 μm)

Fig. 2.4 ...

3 Ependymoma

The tumour cell perikarya are usually arranged in small, closely knit groups with a complex, mosaic-like pattern. These islands of cell bodies are interspersed with larger areas of interlacing processes, which may form a prominent component of the tumour. Typical cells have large nuclei with finely granular chromatin and prominent nucleoli. There is moderately abundant, electron-lucent perikaryal cytoplasm, and most cells contain rather sparse but varied organelles, including randomly orientated 20-nm microtubules and scanty 6- to 9-nm glial filaments. The interlacing cell processes are closely packed together but are not joined by membrane junctions. They are mostly electron lucent and again contain scanty microtubules and glial filaments. The perivascular pseudorosettes seen on light microscopy consist ultrastructurally of a broad zone of these interlacing processes, which extend to envelop closely the outer basement membranes around blood vessels. The vessels themselves have an essentially normal fine structure.

Although many areas lack other, specialised features, the better differentiated tumours also show characteristic intercellular microrosettes. These are formed by two or more adjacent cells joined at their apical surfaces by complexes of zonulae adherentes, zonulae occludens and desmosome junctions. Cross-cut microrosettes may appear entirely intracellular. The lumina are often entirely filled by a meshwork of tightly packed microvilli. Basal bodies (the ultrastructural equivalent of blepharoplasts) are frequently encountered, but cilia are less often seen.

When present, they may project into the lumina of microrosettes, and usually have a normal glial-type configuration of nine peripheral and two central tubules, although abnormal variations occur.

In addition to ependymal-like features, most tumours also contain cell bodies and processes which are almost entirely filled by dense bundles of glial filaments, and have a more astrocytic appearance. These fibrillary elements may predominate in some areas, giving an impression of considerable tumour heterogeneity. Such variation is thought to be the result of a single population of neoplastic glial cells which is recapitulating the various different stages of ependymal embryogenesis, including that of divergent astrocytic specialisation.

Further Reading

Goebel HH, Cravioto H (1972) Ultrastructure of human and experimental ependymomas. J Neuropathol Exp Neurol 31: 55–71

Hirano A, Ghatak NR, Wisoff HS, Zimmerman HM (1971) Comparative ultrastructural study of ependymoma and ependymal cyst. Am J Pathol 62: 11a

Liu HM, McLone DG, Clark S (1977) Ependymomas of childhood. Childs Brain 3: 281–296

Raimondi AJ, Mullan S, Evans JP (1962) Human brain tumours. An electron microscopic study. J Neurosurg 19: 731–753

Tani E, Higashi N (1972) Intercellular junctions in human ependymomas. Acta Neuropathol 22: 295–304

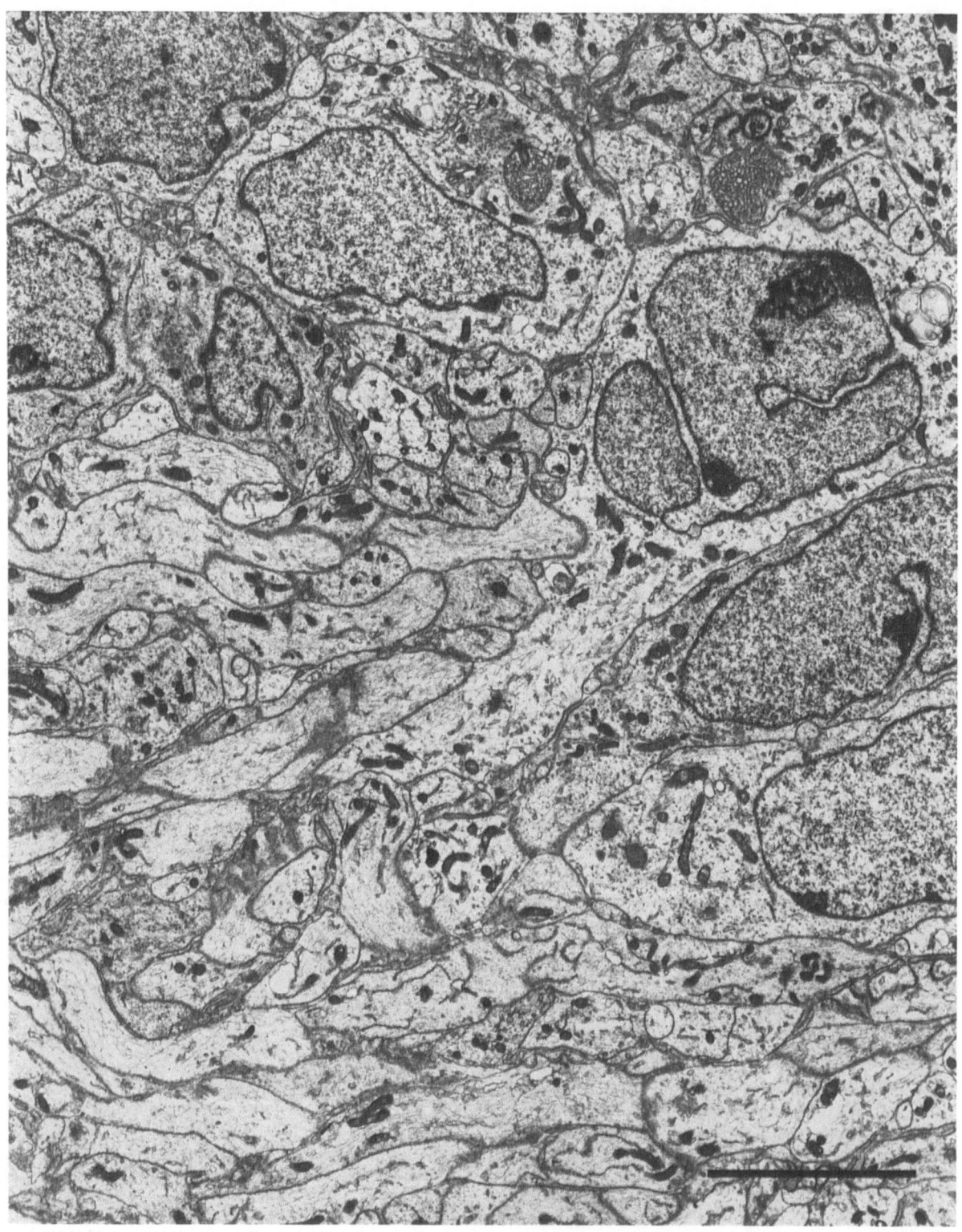

Fig. 3.1. *Ependymoma.* The tumour cell bodies are typically arranged in mosaic-like clumps, as towards the *top* of this figure, and are interspersed with areas of interlacing processes, like those seen in the *lower part* of the field. Cell nuclei are usually large with finely granular chromatin, and there are often prominent nucleoli. (Bar = 5 μm)

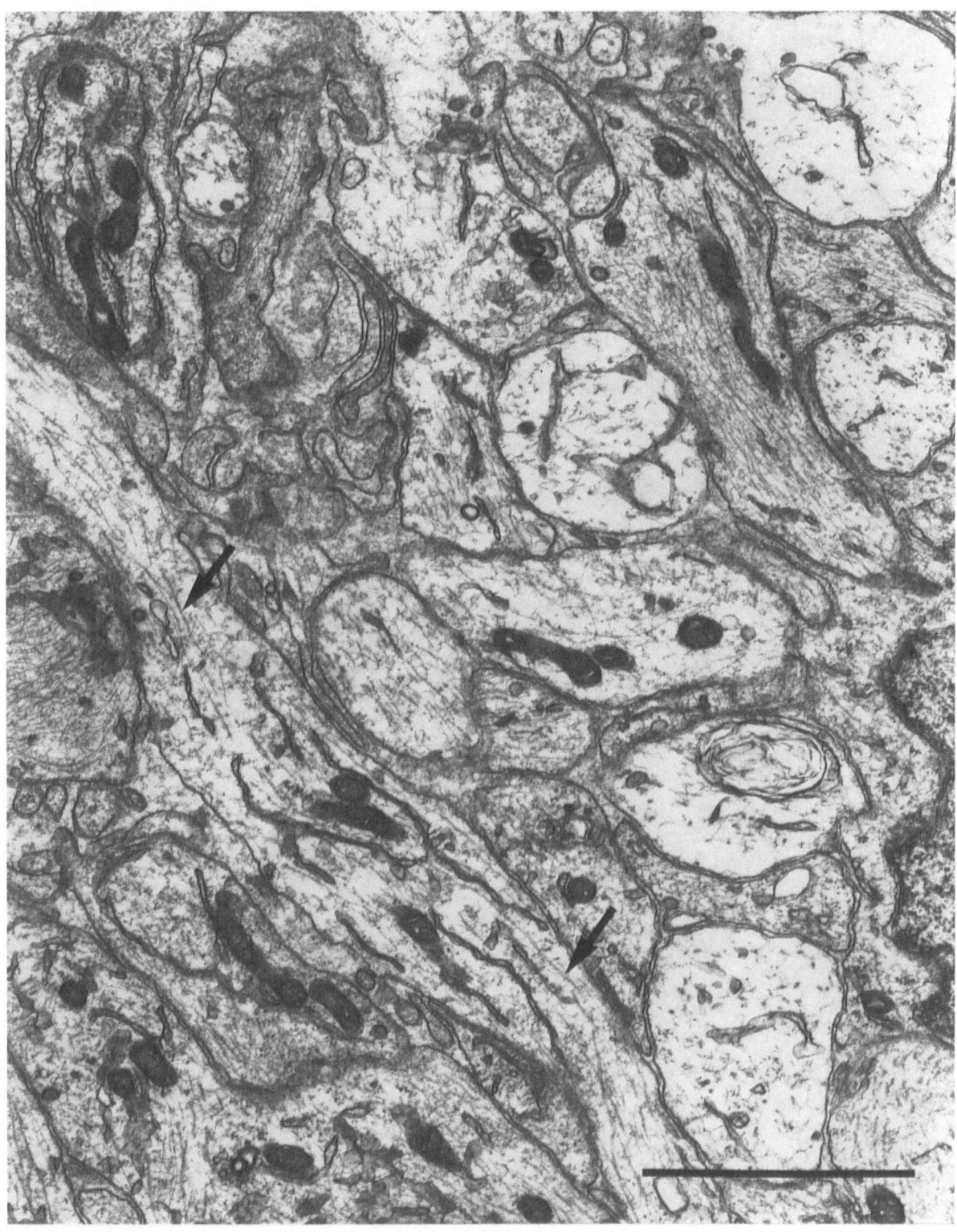

Fig. 3.2. *Ependymoma.* Interlacing, electron-lucent cell processes, like those shown here, are a prominent feature in most of these tumours. The processes usually contain scanty 20-nm microtubules (*arrows*) and 6- to 9-nm glial filaments. Although the processes are tightly packed together in most areas, they lack junctional attachments. (Bar = 2 μm)

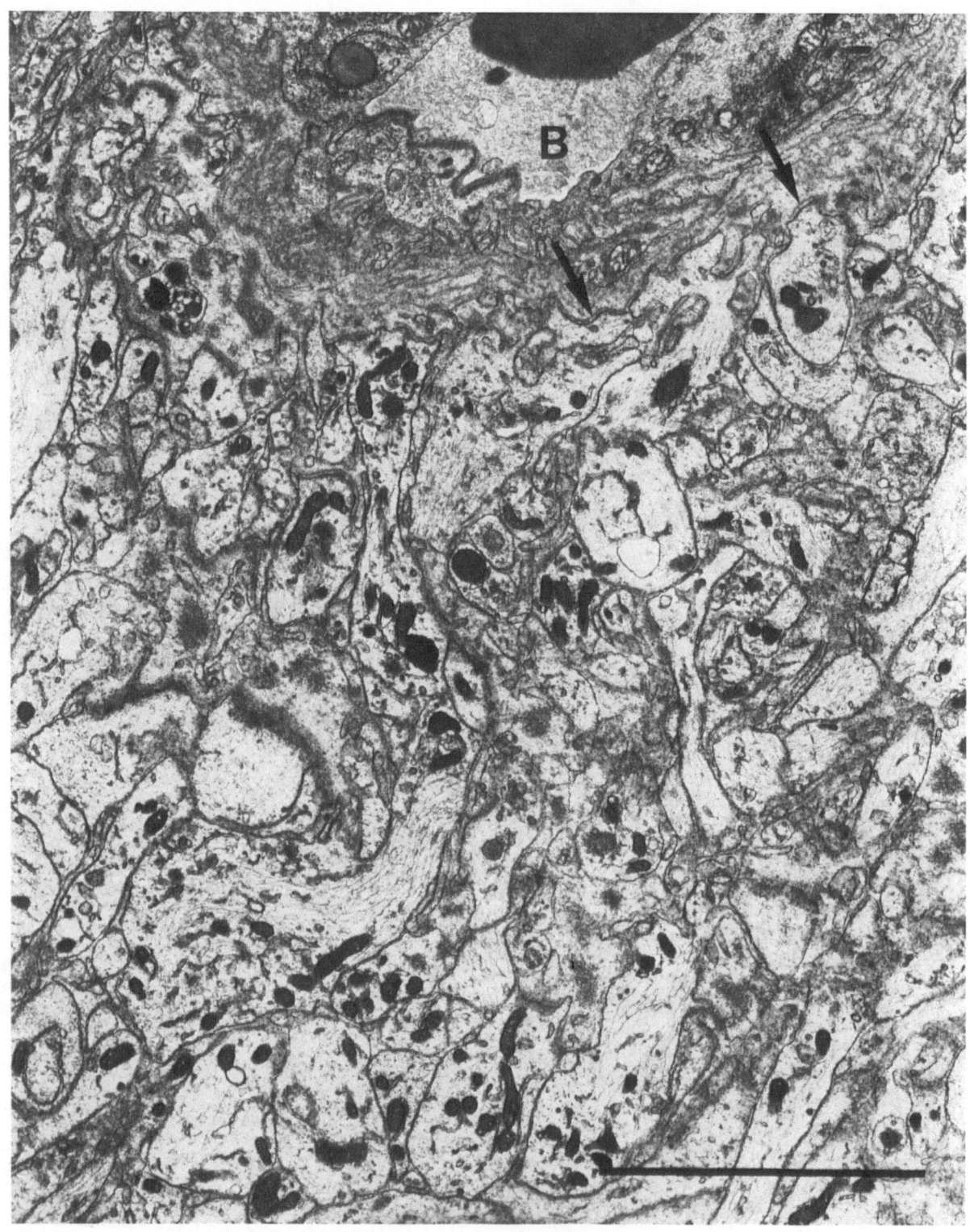

Fig. 3.3. *Ependymoma.* Perivascular pseudorosettes are formed ultrastructurally by a broad zone of interlacing tumour cell processes. This figure shows a small part of such a rosette, with the central blood vessel visible at the *top* (*B*). At the inner margin of the rosette, the meshwork of processes is closely applied to the outer vascular basement membrane (*arrows*). (Bar = 5 μm)

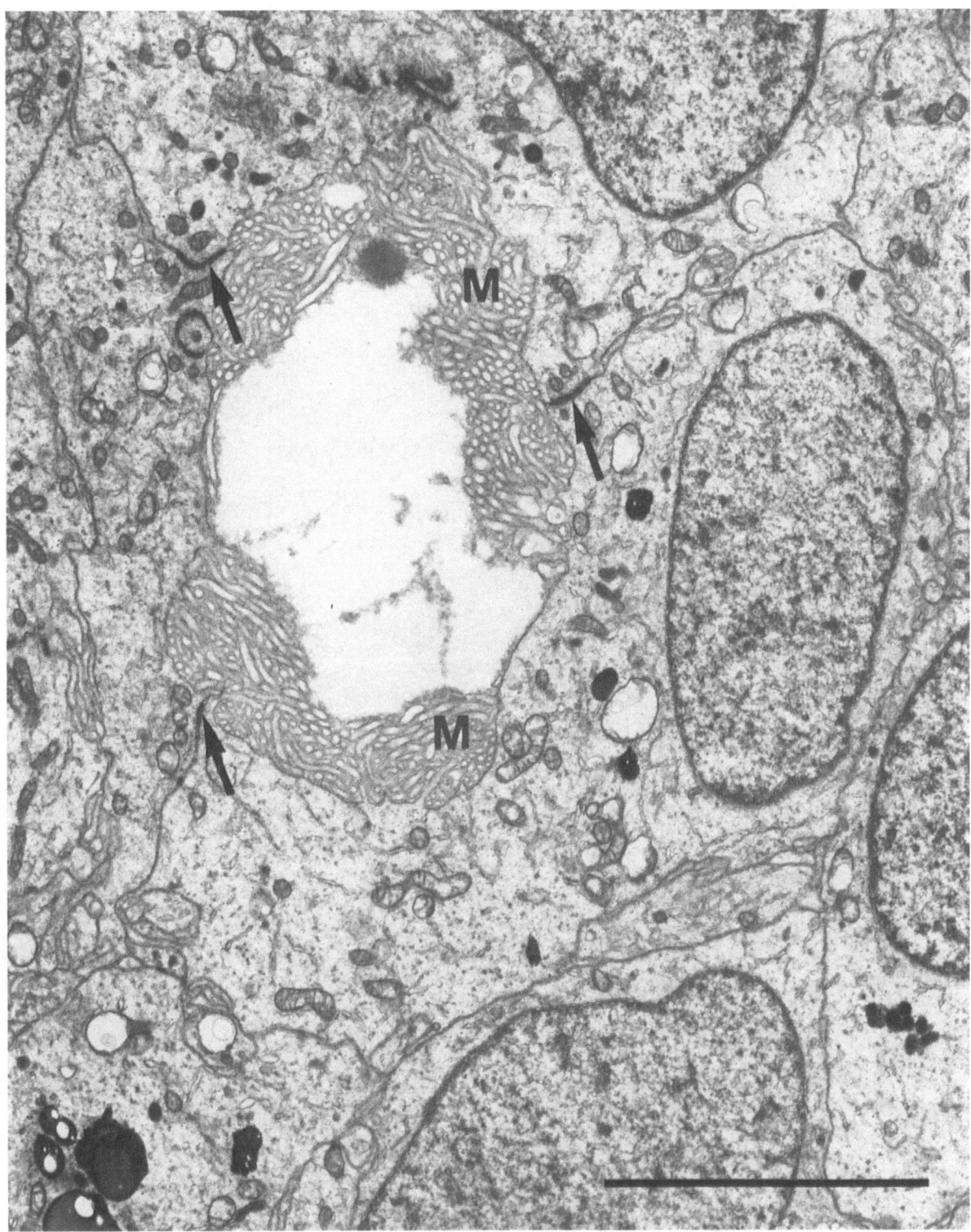

Fig. 3.4. *Ependymoma*. Intercellular microrosettes, like the one shown here, are a distinctive ultrastructural feature of well-differentiated ependymomas. They are formed by two or more adjacent cells, joined at their apical surfaces by junctional complexes (*arrows*), and their lumina usually contain abundant microvilli (*M*). The tumour cells in this picture are typical of ependymoma cells, and have moderately abundant, electron-lucent cytoplasm containing sparse but varied organelles. (Bar = 5 μm)

21

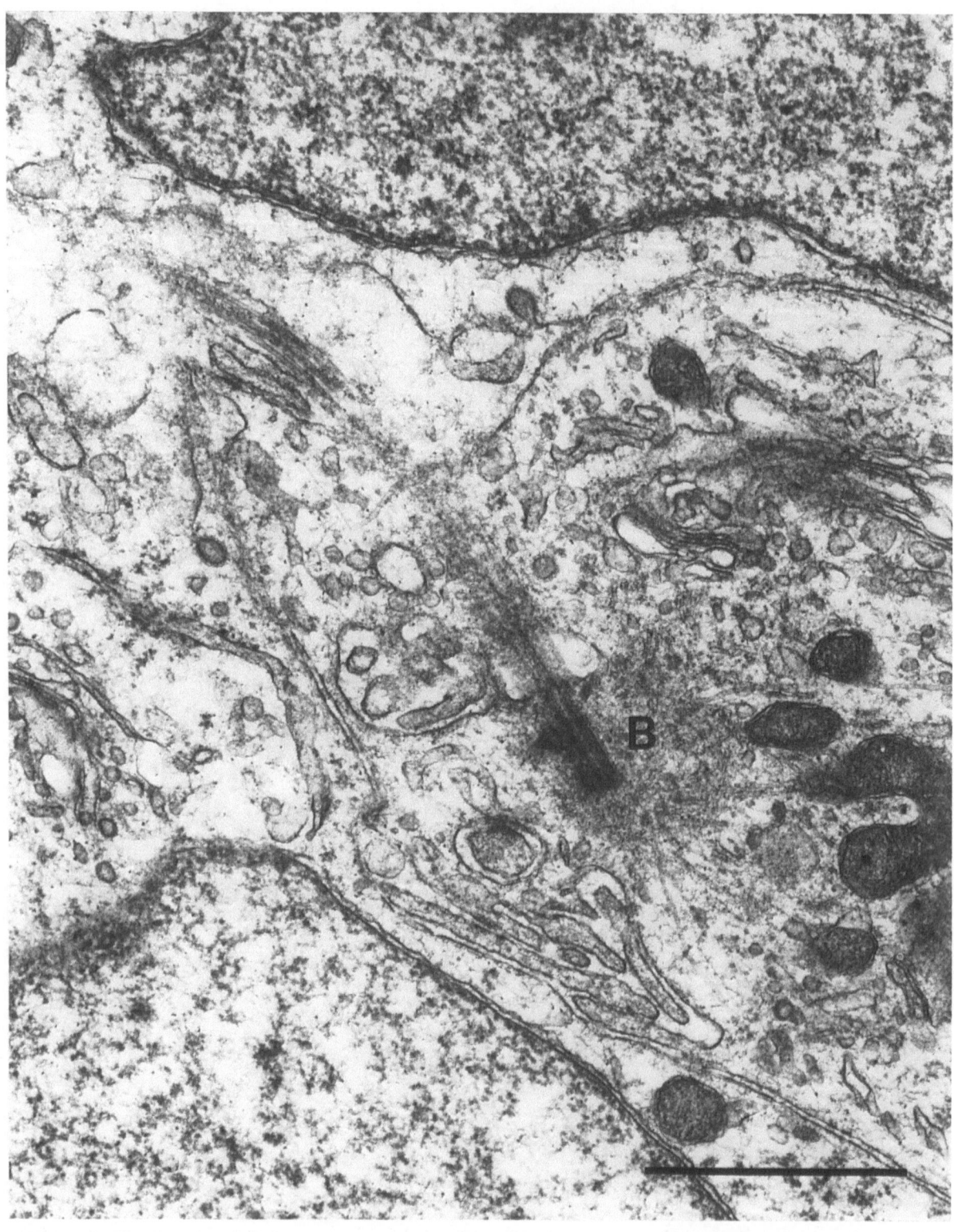

Fig. 3.5. *Ependymoma.* Cilia projecting from tumour cell bodies may appear isolated, as in this example, or occur as small clusters. In some instances they project into the lumina of intercellular microrosettes. The blepharoplasts seen at light microscopic level are formed from the basal bodies of cilia (*B*). (Bar = 1 µm)

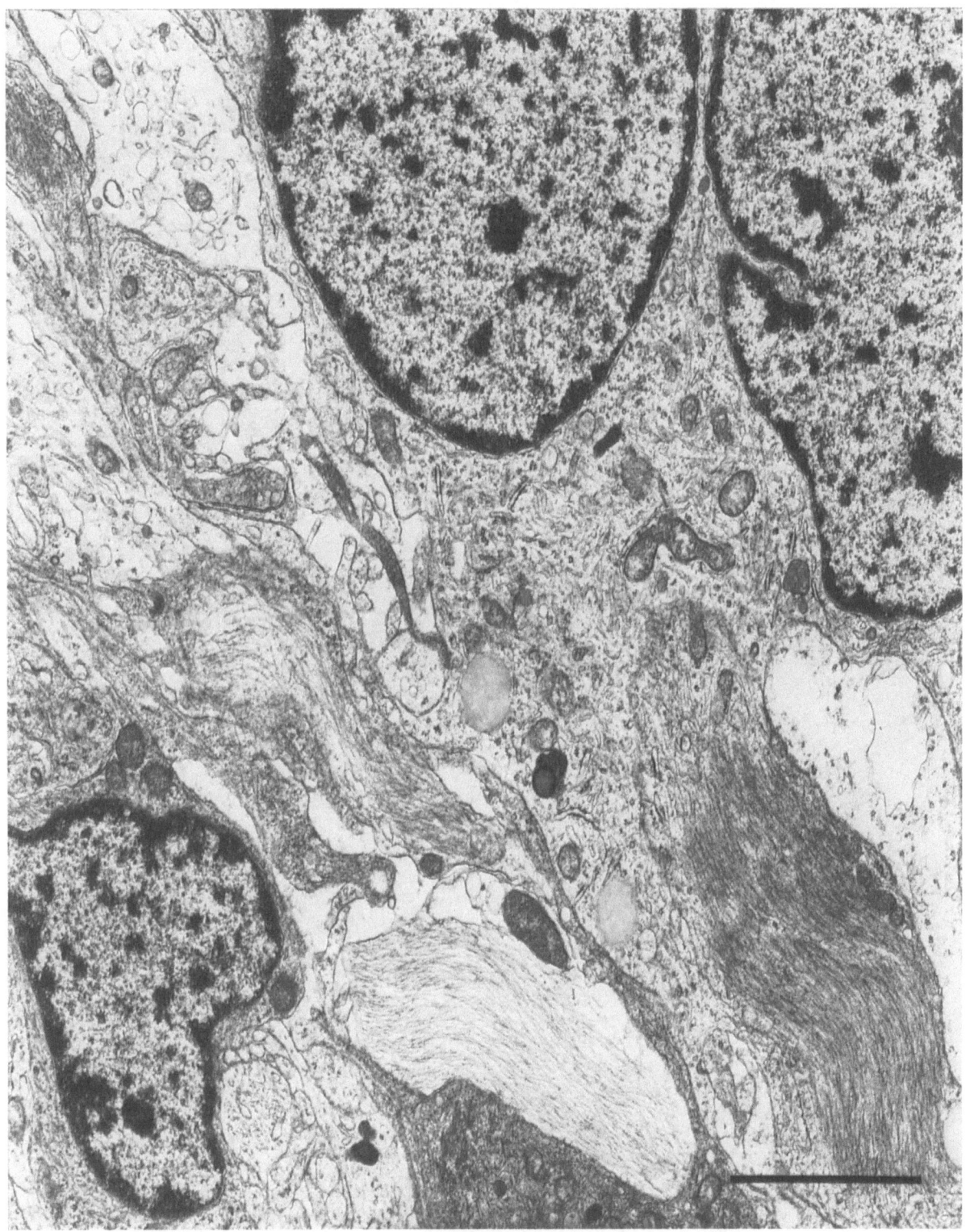

Fig. 3.6. *Ependymoma.* Most tumours contain some astrocytic-type tumour cells and processes, like those shown here, which are filled with dense bundles of 6- to 9-nm glial filaments. Although such astrocytic elements are often sparsely distributed, in some ependymomas there may be areas where they are a prominent feature. (Bar = 2 μm)

4 Myxopapillary Ependymoma

Myxopapillary ependymomas represent a variant of ependymoma, and the ultrastructural appearance in some areas may be typically ependymomatous, with tightly packed cell processes and mosaic-like groups of tumour cells forming ependymal microrosettes. In many areas, however, the tumour cells have a more irregular, stellate appearance, with long tenuous processes separated by abundant extracellular space. Glial filaments are present in both the processes and cell bodies, and may be a prominent feature in some cells. The expanded extracellular space is lined by continuous basement membrane and contains scattered collagen fibres mixed with amorphous or finely fibrillar material. Smaller loculi of extracellular space are enclosed by a loose meshwork of tumour cell processes, but larger areas may be lined by uniformly orientated tumour cell bodies, with apical junctional complexes (including zonulae occludens and desmosomes) and prominent clumps of apical microvilli. Such appearances are reminiscent of choroid plexus tissue, which has a common embryological origin with ependymal cells. Like the other extracellular spaces within the tumour, the perivascular spaces are also markedly enlarged. They again contain scanty collagen fibres mixed with amorphous material, and are lined by intact basement membrane. In all areas, the tumour basement membrane is abnormally thickened and often shows three distinct layers. The loose, inner zone and central, compact region are narrow and well defined, but the outer zone is broad and irregular, often merging with the amorphous material in the extracellular space. This material probably represents the myxoid ground substance visible on light microscopy, and appears to be formed by the abnormal proliferation of tumour cell basement membrane. There is experimental evidence that collagen fibres may stimulate basement membrane production, and it has been suggested that a similar mechanism operates in the myxopapillary ependymomas of the cauda equina, where collagen is normally found in close relation to non-neoplastic ependymal cells.

Further Reading

Liu HM, McLone DG, Clark S (1977) Ependymomas of childhood. Childs Brain 3: 281–296
Rawlinson DG, Herman MM, Rubinstein LJ (1973) The fine structure of a myxopapillary ependymoma of the filum terminale. Acta Neuropathol 25: 1–13

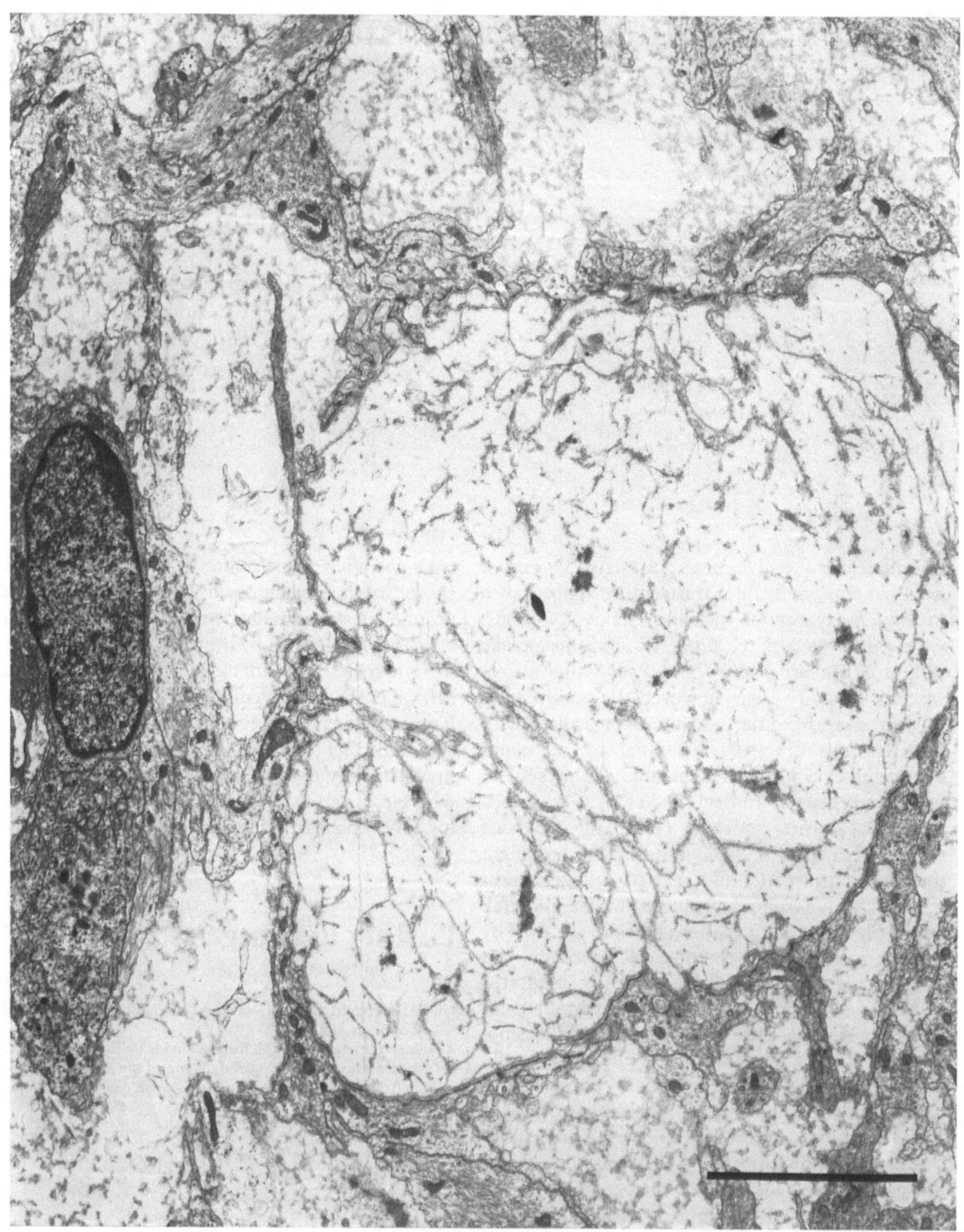

Fig. 4.1. *Myxopapillary ependymoma.* In many areas the extracellular space is greatly expanded and divided into separate pockets, or loculi, like the one filling the *centre* of this figure. These loculi are enclosed by a loose meshwork of cell processes and lined by basement membrane. Isolated tumour cell bodies, like that seen on the *left*, are widely separated and have an irregular outline. (Bar = 5 μm)

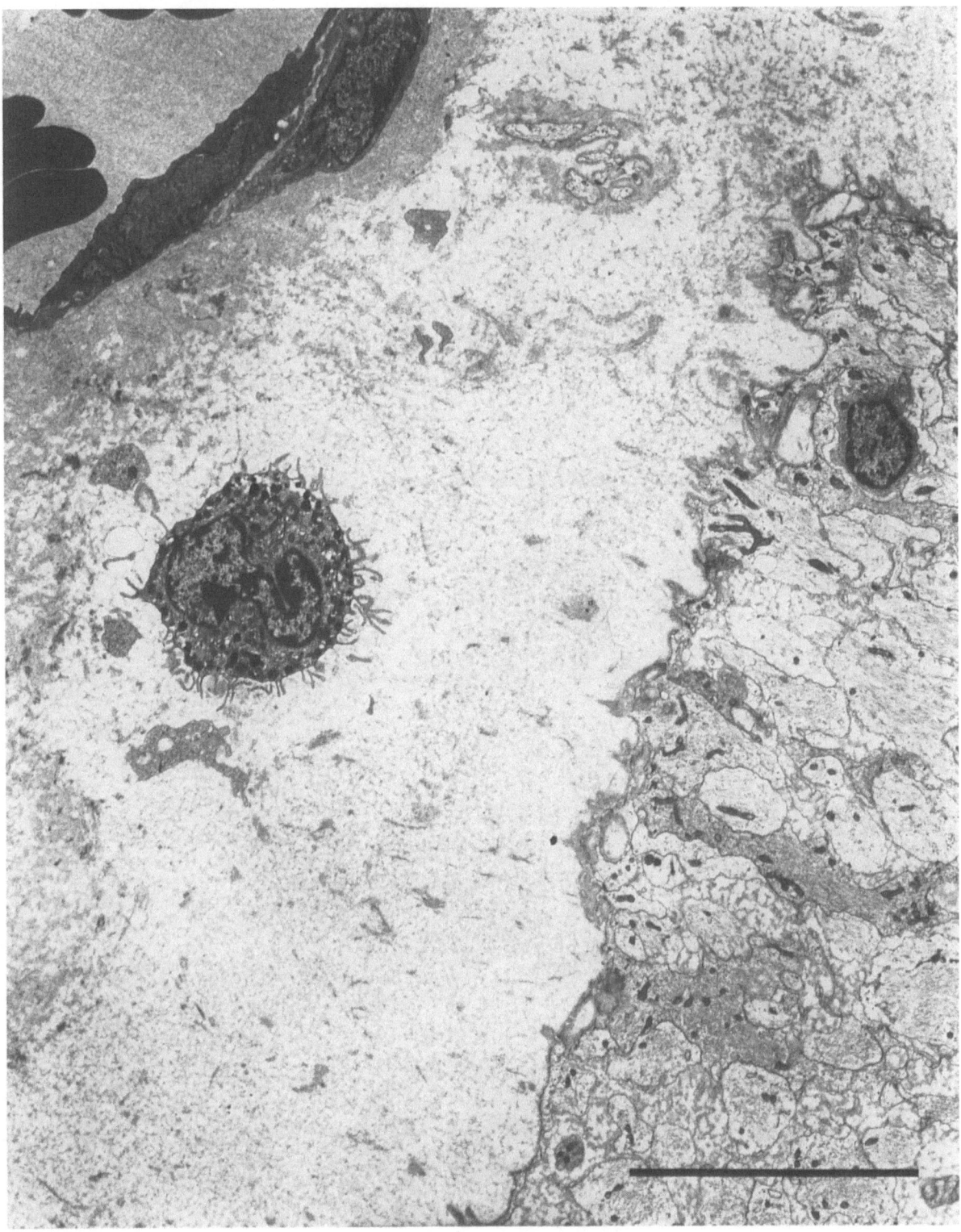

Fig. 4.2. *Myxopapillary ependymoma.* Around blood vessels (*top left corner*), the cell processes may be more closely packed together, as seen on the *right*. The perivascular spaces are lined by outer basement membrane and are often abnormally wide, like the one shown here. They usually contain only very scanty collagen and amorphous material, but in this case a mast cell is also present. (Bar = 10 μm)

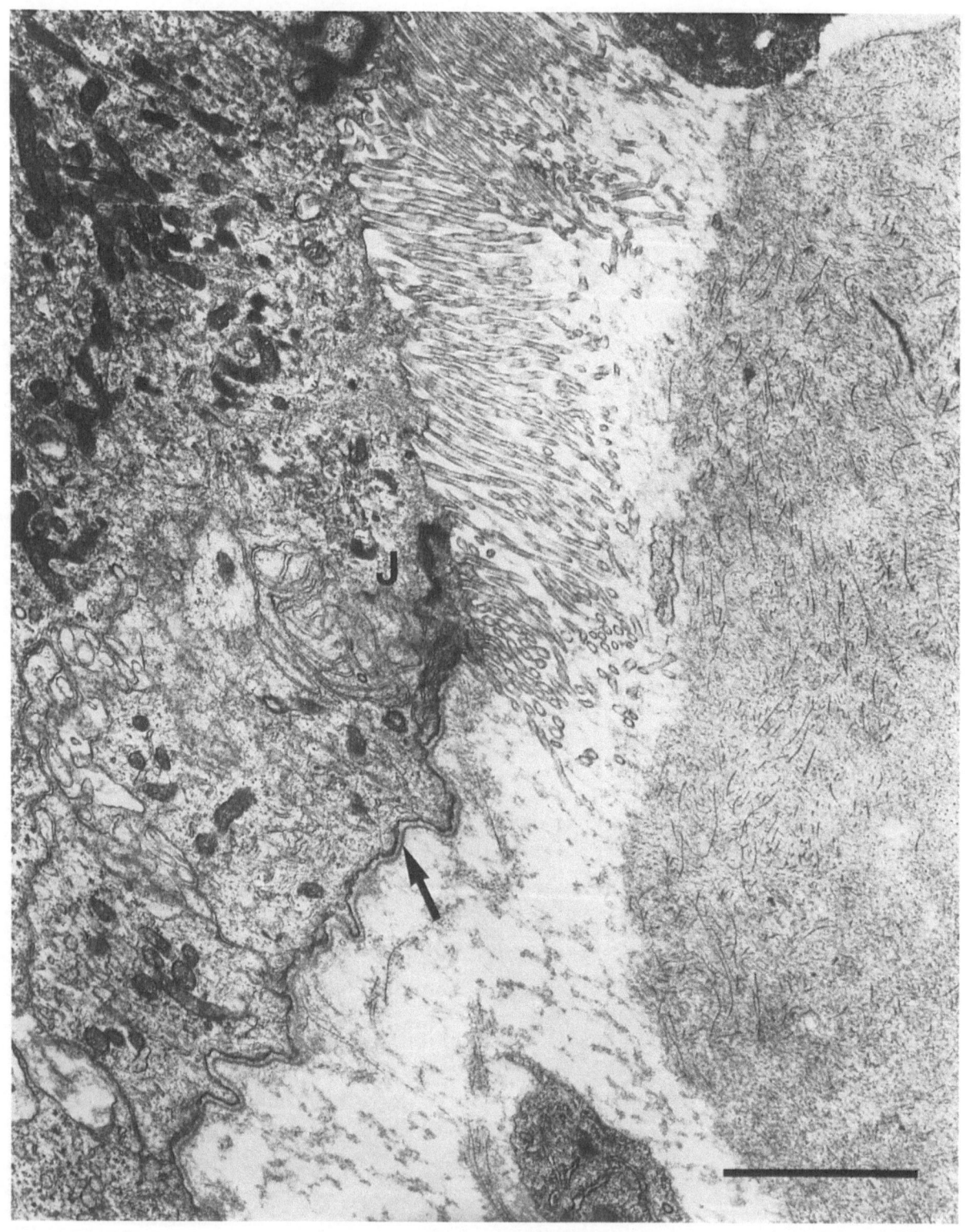

Fig. 4.3. *Myxopapillary ependymoma.* Larger areas of extracellular space may be lined by palisades of tumour cell bodies joined by apical junctional complexes (*J*). These cells are usually covered by basement membrane (*arrow*), but as in the *upper part* of this field, there may also be prominent apical microvilli, giving an appearance reminiscent of choroid plexus tissue. The extracellular space contains abundant fibrillary and amorphous material, visible on the *right*. (Bar = 2 μm)

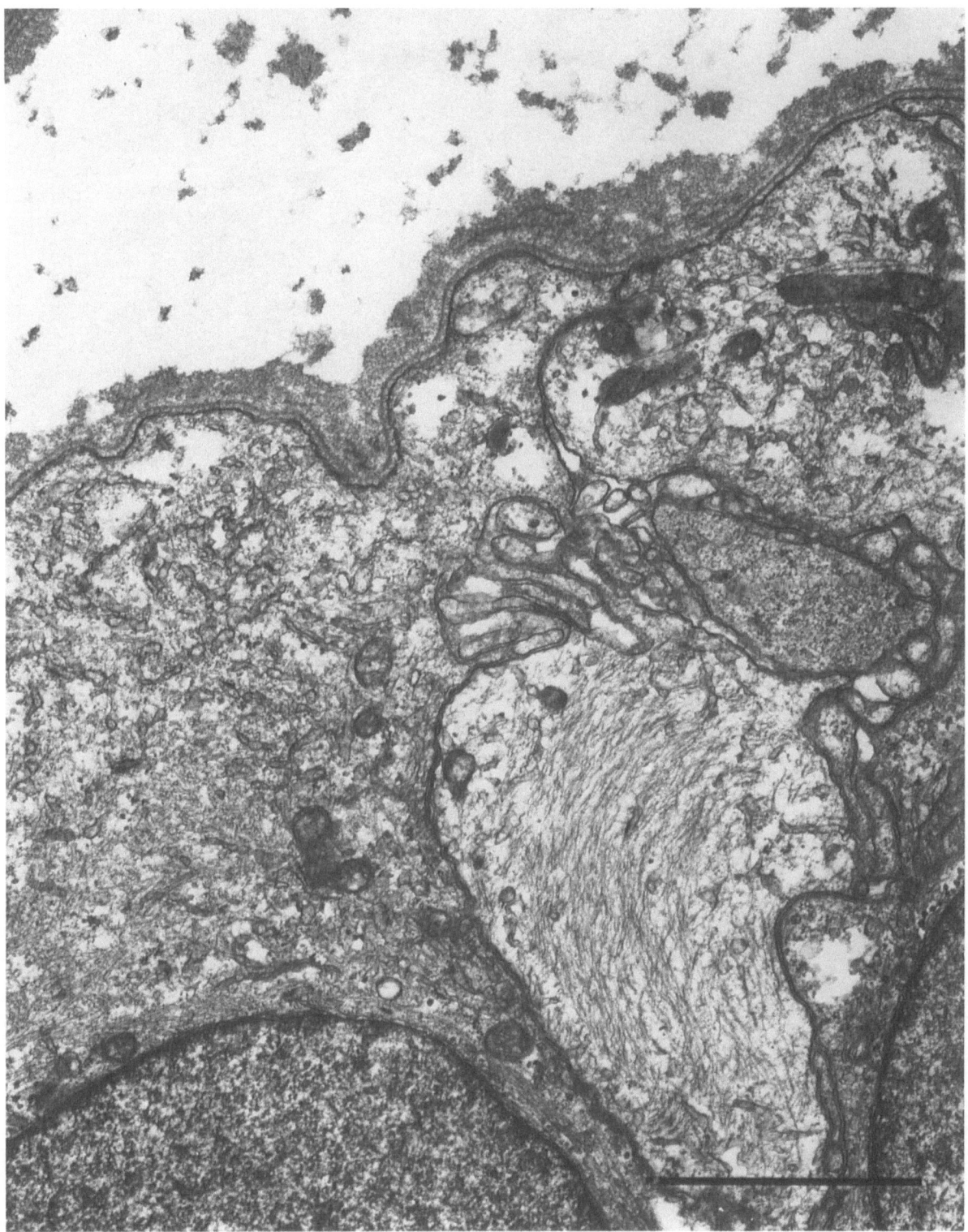

Fig. 4.4. *Myxopapillary ependymoma.* The most distinctive feature of this tumour is the abnormal proliferation of basement membranes. These separate the tumour cells from perivascular and other extracellular spaces and often have three distinct zones, like the one seen at the *top* of this figure. The broad, irregular outer zone may be the source of the amorphous "myxoid" material present in the extracellular spaces. The tumour cells and processes contain variable amounts of 6- to 9-nm glial filaments, as can be seen in the *lower part* of this field. (Bar = 2 μm)

5 Subependymoma

At ultrastructural level subependymomas appear to be distinct from true ependymomas, and consistently show a number of different features. Tumour cell bodies are only loosely grouped together in small clusters, and are widely separated by extensive areas of cell processes which form the bulk of the tumour. The predominant cell has a rather primitive appearance, with a large rounded nucleus and scanty perinuclear cytoplasm. This contains mainly polyribosomes and lacks true peripheral processes. Very occasionally, however, these cells have microvilli projecting from the surface, which may be loosely enclosed into separate pockets by the processes of other adjacent cells and associated zonulae adherentes junctions. Junctional complexes with desmosomes and zonulae occludens are not present, and there are no typical ependymal-type microrosettes. Isolated cilia are very rarely seen, and are usually buried within tumour cell bodies. Other cells present resemble fibrillary astrocytes, with irregular nuclear outlines, clumped chromatin and more abundant cytoplasm which is almost entirely filled by dense bundles of 6- to 9-nm glial filaments. There is apparently a spectrum between these astrocytic cells and the more primitive-looking, ependymal type, and intermediate forms with both filaments and microvilli may sometimes be encountered. The astrocytic cells give rise to the abundant, tightly interlacing cell processes, which are also packed with glial filaments. The astrocytic element is much more pronounced than in typical ependymoma, and in contrast to that tumour, the cell processes in subependymoma are joined by frequent gap junctions and zonulae adherentes. Unlike true astrocytomas, however, virtually no extracellular space is visible between the cell processes, and there is no tendency to form terminal foot processes around blood vessel basement membranes.

There is some debate as to whether this is a primary astrocytic tumour with non-neoplastic ependymal inclusions, or a primary ependymal tumour with pronounced astrocytic differentiation. It has also been suggested that the tumour may arise from relatively undifferentiated ependymoglial precursor cells which persist in the subependymal region and have retained the capacity for both astrocytic and ependymal differentiation.

Further Reading

Azzarelli B, Rekate HL, Roessmann U (1977) Subependymoma. A case report with ultrastructural study. Acta Neuropathol 40: 279–282

Duffell D, Farber L, Chou S, Hartmann JF, Nelson F (1963) Electron microscopic observations on astrocytomas. Subependymal glomerulate astrocytoma. Am J Pathol 43: 539–545

Fu YS, Chen ATL, Kay S, Young HF (1974) Is subependymoma (subependymal glomerulate astrocytoma) an astrocytoma or an ependymoma? A comparative ultrastructural and tissue culture study. Cancer 34: 1992–2008

Moss TH (1984) Observations on the nature of subependymoma. An electron microscopic study. Neuropathol Appl Neurobiol 10: 63–75

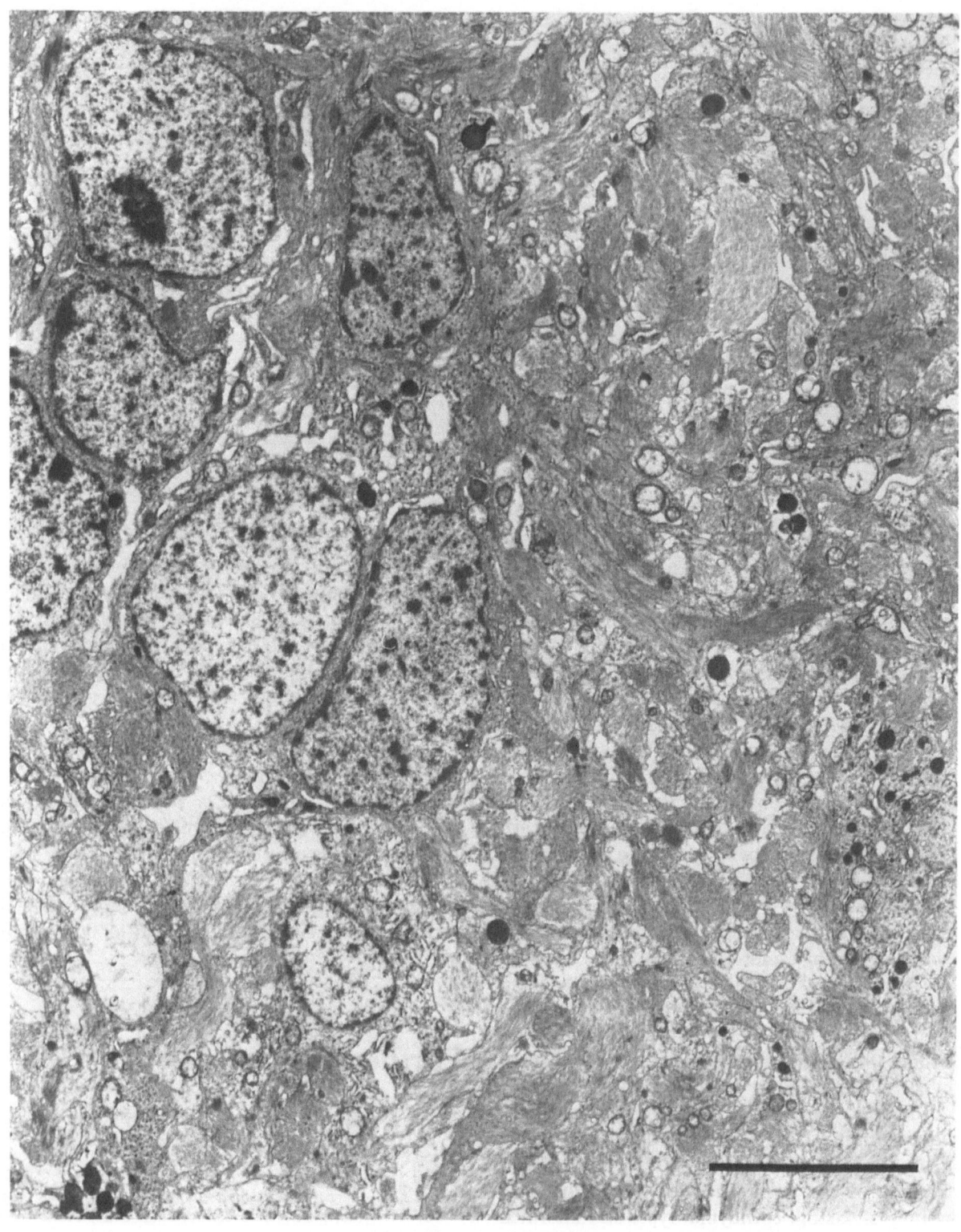

Fig. 5.1. *Subependymoma*. The tumour cells are rather loosely aggregated into small clusters, like that seen on the *left*. They are separated by extensive areas of interlacing cell processes, which constitute the bulk of the tumour tissue. (Bar = 5 μm) (Moss 1984)

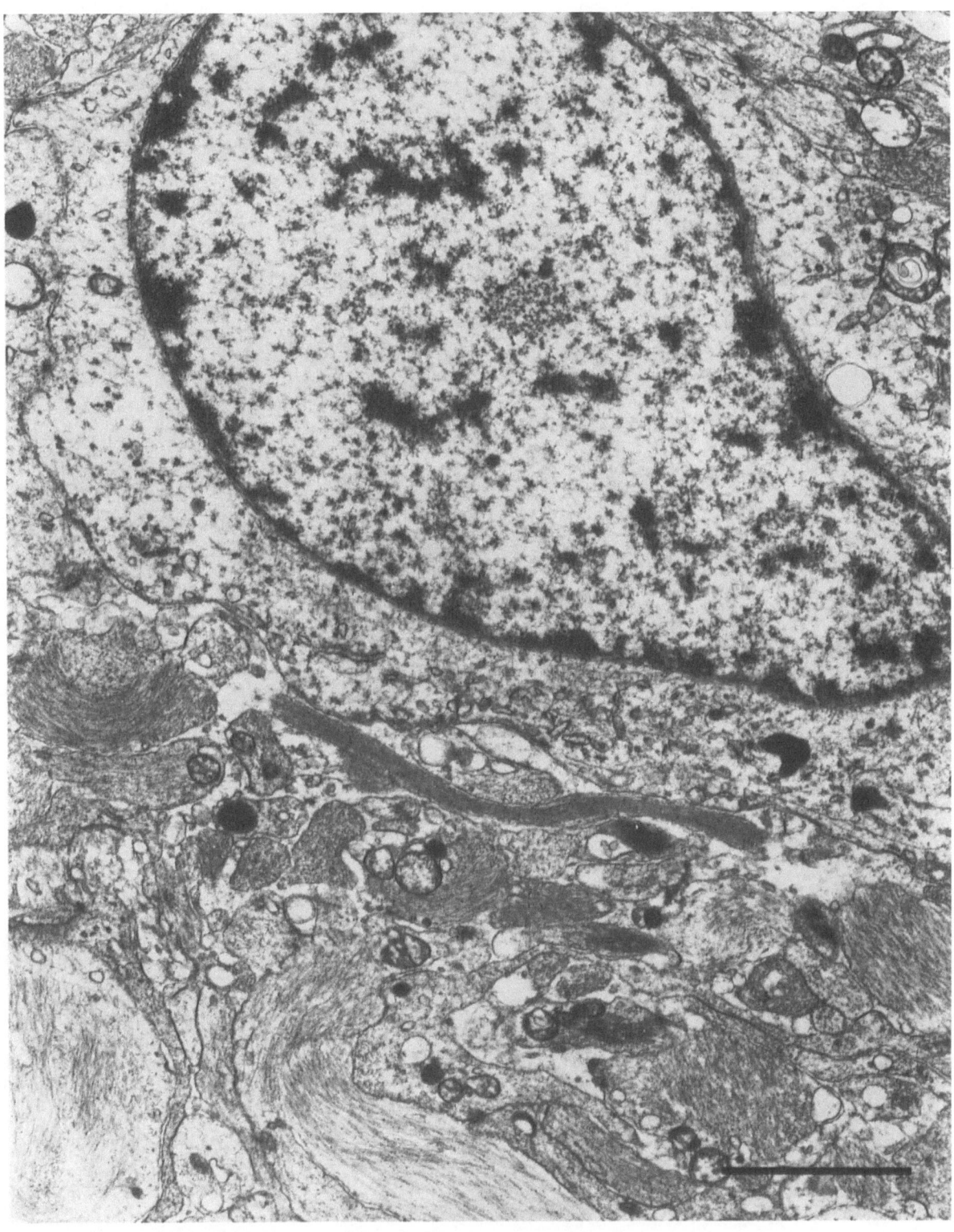

Fig. 5.2. *Subependymoma.* The predominant cell type appears rather primitive, and has a large rounded nucleus but only scanty perinuclear cytoplasm. The cytoplasm contains mainly polyribosomes and shows no tendency to form peripheral processes. These tumour cells may be derived from ependymoglial precursor cells which persist in the subependymal region into adult life and then undergo neoplastic change. (Bar = 2 μm) (Moss 1984)

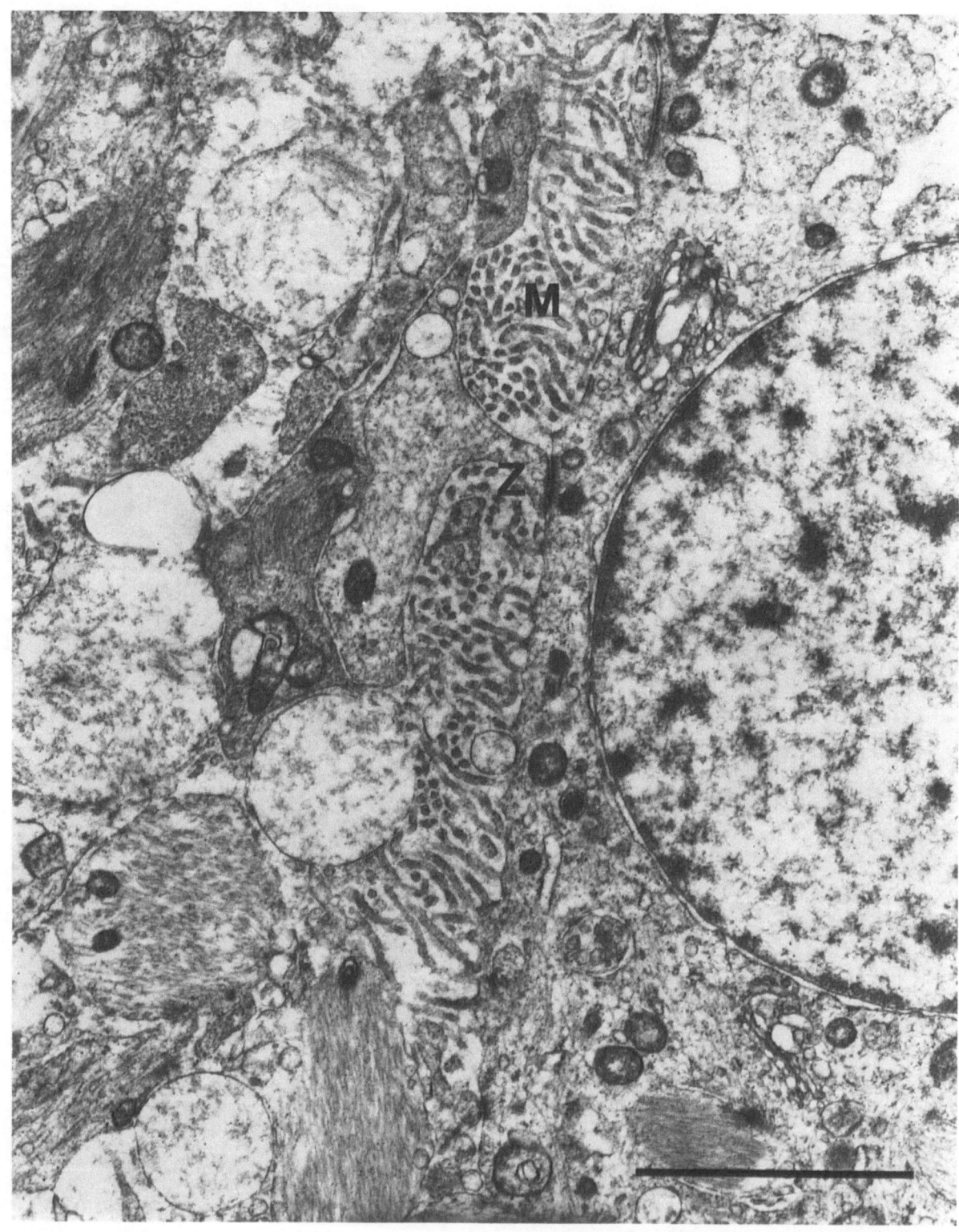

Fig. 5.3. *Subependymoma.* Occasional cells have surface microvilli (*M*), as in the example shown here. The microvilli may be loosely enclosed into separate pockets by the processes of adjacent cells and associated isolated zonulae adherentes junctions (Z). Junctional complexes with desmosomes are not present, and typical ependymal microrosettes are not a feature of these tumours. (Bar = 2 μm) (Moss 1984)

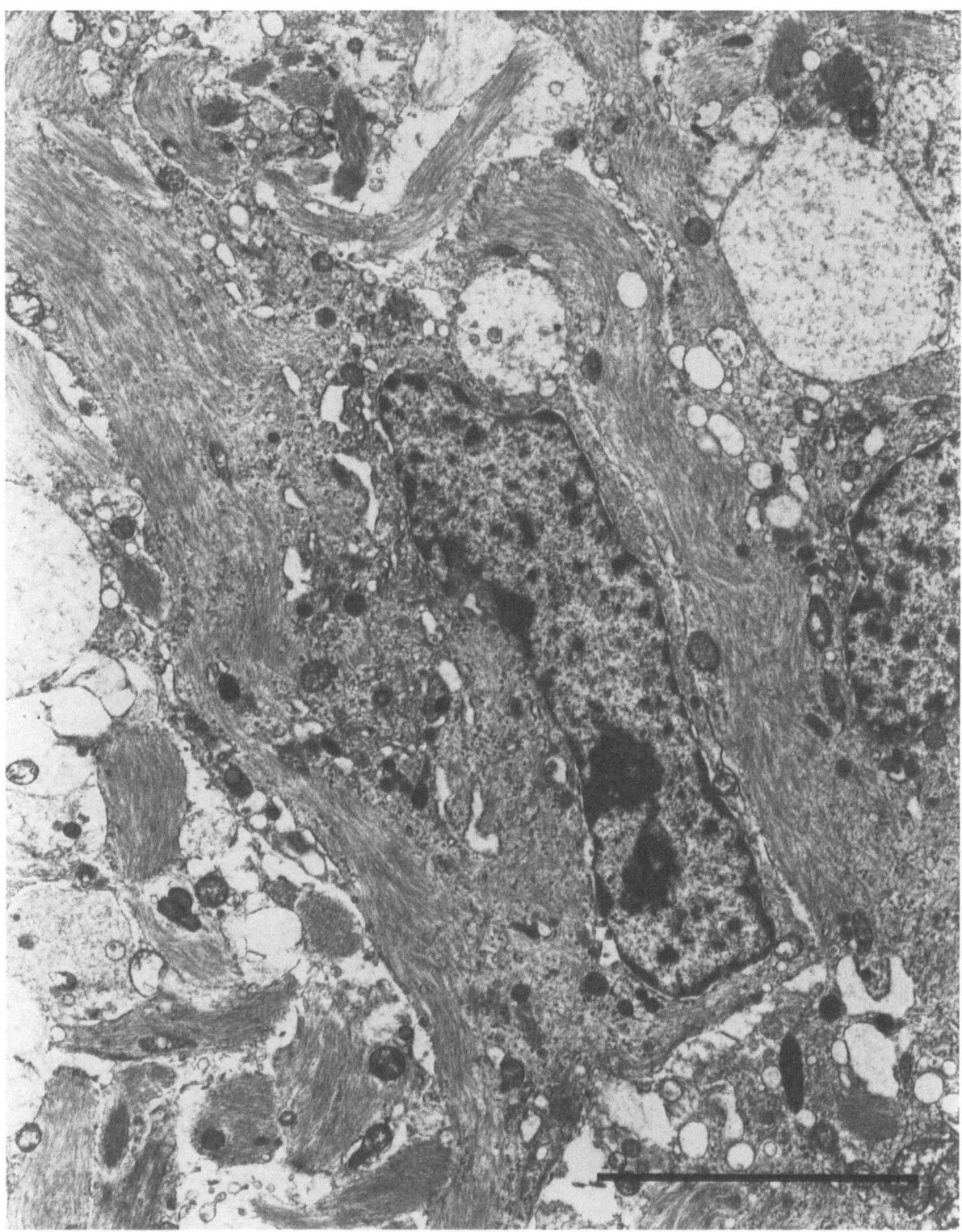

Fig. 5.4. *Subependymoma.* A second, apparently distinct cell type is illustrated here and resembles a fibrillary astrocyte. These cells have irregular nuclei and abundant cytoplasm filled by dense bundles of 6- to 9-nm glial filaments. They give rise to the abundant, interlacing cell processes which are typical of subependymomas. Intermediate forms of cell showing both microvilli and abundant filaments may also be seen in some cases. (Bar = 5 μm) (Moss 1984)

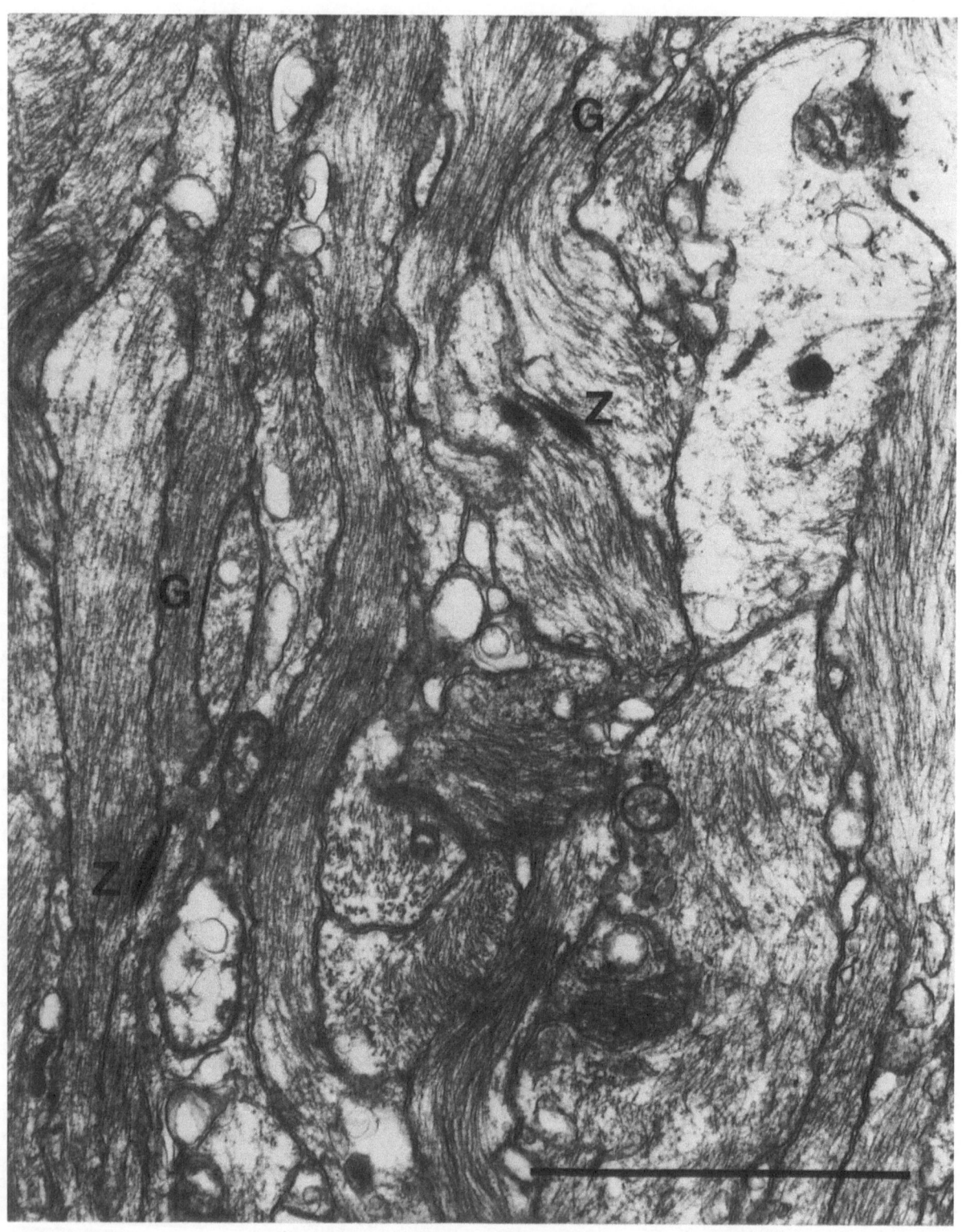

Fig. 5.5. *Subependymoma.* The cell processes constituting the bulk of these tumours are packed with 6- to 9-nm glial filaments. Unlike the cell processes in ependymomas, they are joined by numerous gap junctions (G) and zonulae adherentes (Z). In contrast to astrocytomas, there is no visible extracellular space and no tendency to form foot processes around vascular basement membranes. (Bar = 2 μm) (Moss 1984)

6 Malignant Glioma

The term malignant glioma is used here to describe malignant tumours of glial origin in which the lack of differentiation at ultrastructural level precludes recognition of specific astrocytic, oligodendroglial or ependymal features. In all cases a glial origin can be established by the presence of bundles of 6- to 9-nm glial-type filaments. Although many of these neoplasms probably derive from malignant astrocytes rather than other glial types, they are ultrastructurally distinct from the non-malignant types of astrocytoma. Many attempts to grade the cell types in malignant glioma have been made on the basis of their varied ultrastructural appearances, but such subclassification is not generally regarded as useful because of the numerous transitional forms present in any grading system.

In more central areas, away from the infiltrating margins, these neoplasms usually have a solid appearance, with numerous and closely packed tumour cell perikarya. In contrast to astrocytomas, little or no extracellular space is visible between adjacent cells. Nuclei are generally large with an irregular outline, and there is often a prominent nucleolus. Mitotic figures are present in some cells, with dissolution of the nuclear membrane and distinctive aggregation of chromatin. Perinuclear cytoplasm is often rather scanty, and contains generally sparse organelles but abundant polyribosomes. Bundles of glial filaments are a very variable feature, and moderately well-differentiated astrocytic cells containing prominent bundles of filaments may be found alongside tumour cells entirely devoid of filaments. In general, the degree of gliofibrillar differentiation is more apparent than by light microscopy in all these tumours, but in some cases glial filaments are scarce and confined to wispy bundles in a very few cells. Cell processes, which may be present between some of the cell bodies, are more likely to contain filaments than the perikaryal cytoplasm.

Blood vessels are often abnormally hyperplastic, and the swollen, proliferated endothelial cells frequently obliterate the narrowed vascular lumina. Larger vessels also show proliferation of pericytes and striking reduplication of surrounding basement membrane. In addition, there may be abnormally abundant perivascular collagen, with associated fibroblastic spindle cells.

In glioblastoma multiforme the ultrastructural appearances are similar to those of other malignant gliomas, but in some areas the cells may show considerable pleomorphism, with bizarre or multiple nuclei and voluminous cytoplasm. The configuration and organelle content of these cells is very variable and there is often a prominent ruffling or redundancy of the plasma membranes, sometimes amounting to microvillous formation. Glial filaments are usually very scanty, and may be entirely absent in the majority of the more pleomorphic cells.

Further Reading

Hess JR (1978) Frequency of surface microprojections and coated vesicles with increased malignancy in human astrocytic neoplasms. Acta Neuropathol 44: 151–153

Hossman KA, Wechsler W (1971) Ultrastructural cytopathology of human cerebral gliomas. Oncology 26: 455–480

Jellinger K (1978) Glioblastoma multiforme: morphology and biology. Acta Neurochir (Wein) 42: 5–32

Luse SA (1960) Electron microscopic studies of brain tumours. Neurology 10: 881–905

Zülch KJ, Wechsler W (1968) Pathology and classification of gliomas. In: Kragenbuhl H, Maspes PE, Sweet WH (eds) Neurological surgery, vol 2. Karger, Basel, pp 1–84

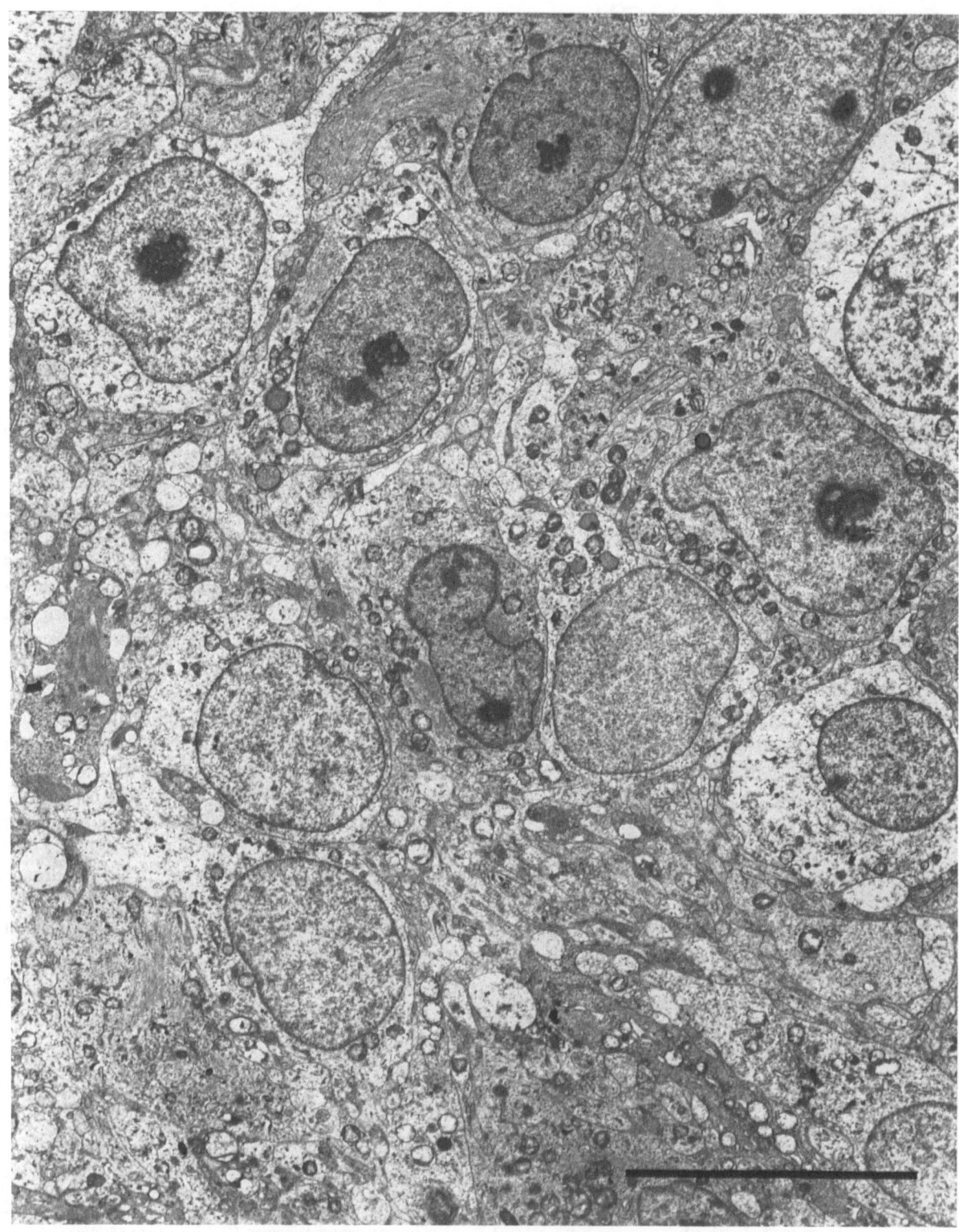

Fig. 6.1. *Malignant glioma.* In the solid, more central areas, tumour cell bodies are usually closely packed together in sheets, with occasional intervening cell processes. In contrast to typical astrocytomas, there is little free extracellular space. The cell nuclei are irregular with frequent nucleoli and the perikaryal cytoplasm is often rather scanty. (Bar = 10 μm)

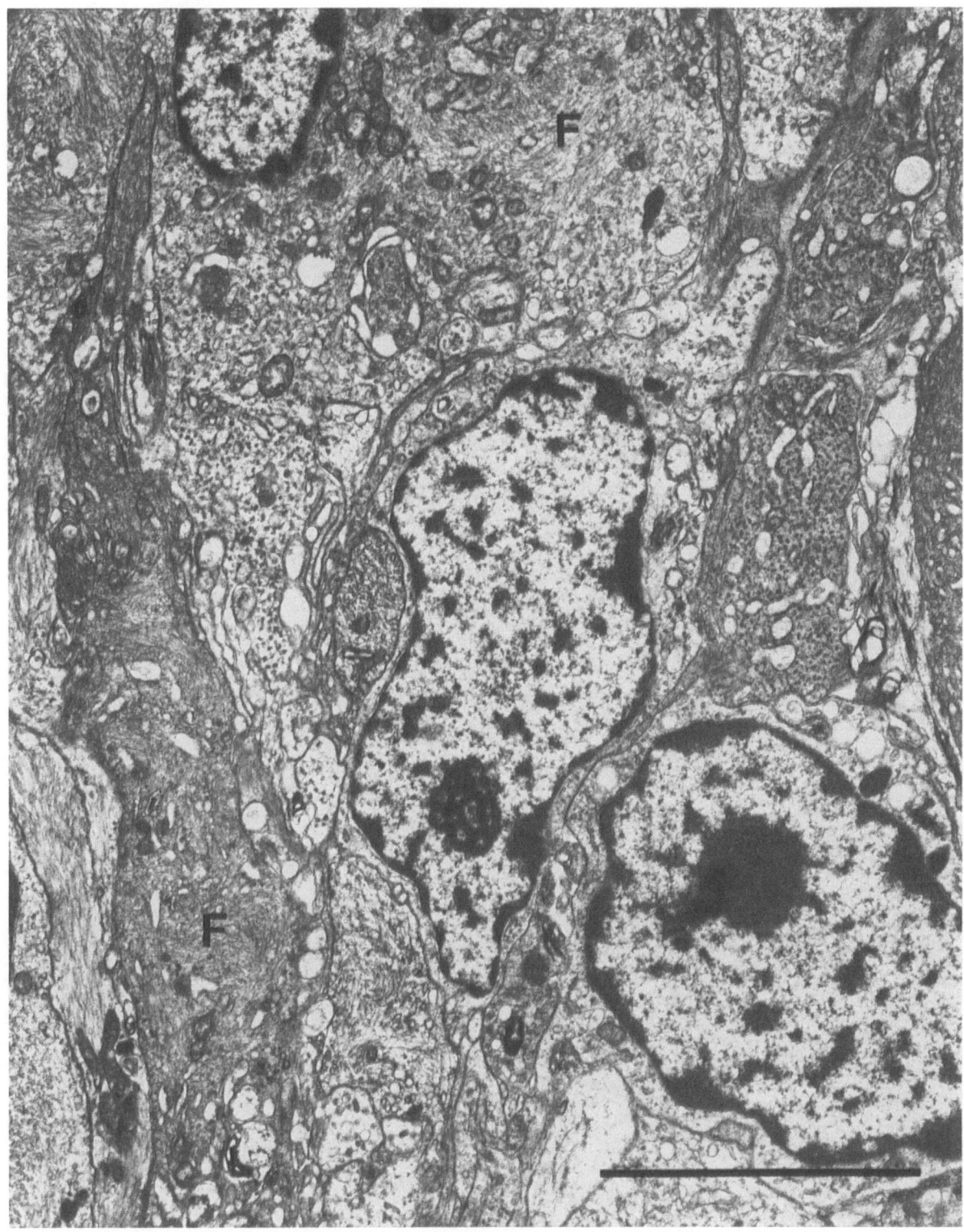

Fig. 6.2. *Malignant glioma.* The cytoplasm of tumour cells typically contains rather sparse organelles but there may be abundant polyribosomes. As in the area shown here, bundles of 6- to 9-nm glial filaments (*F*) can usually be found in at least some of the cells, although more often in their processes than in the perikaryal cytoplasm. (Bar = 5 μm)

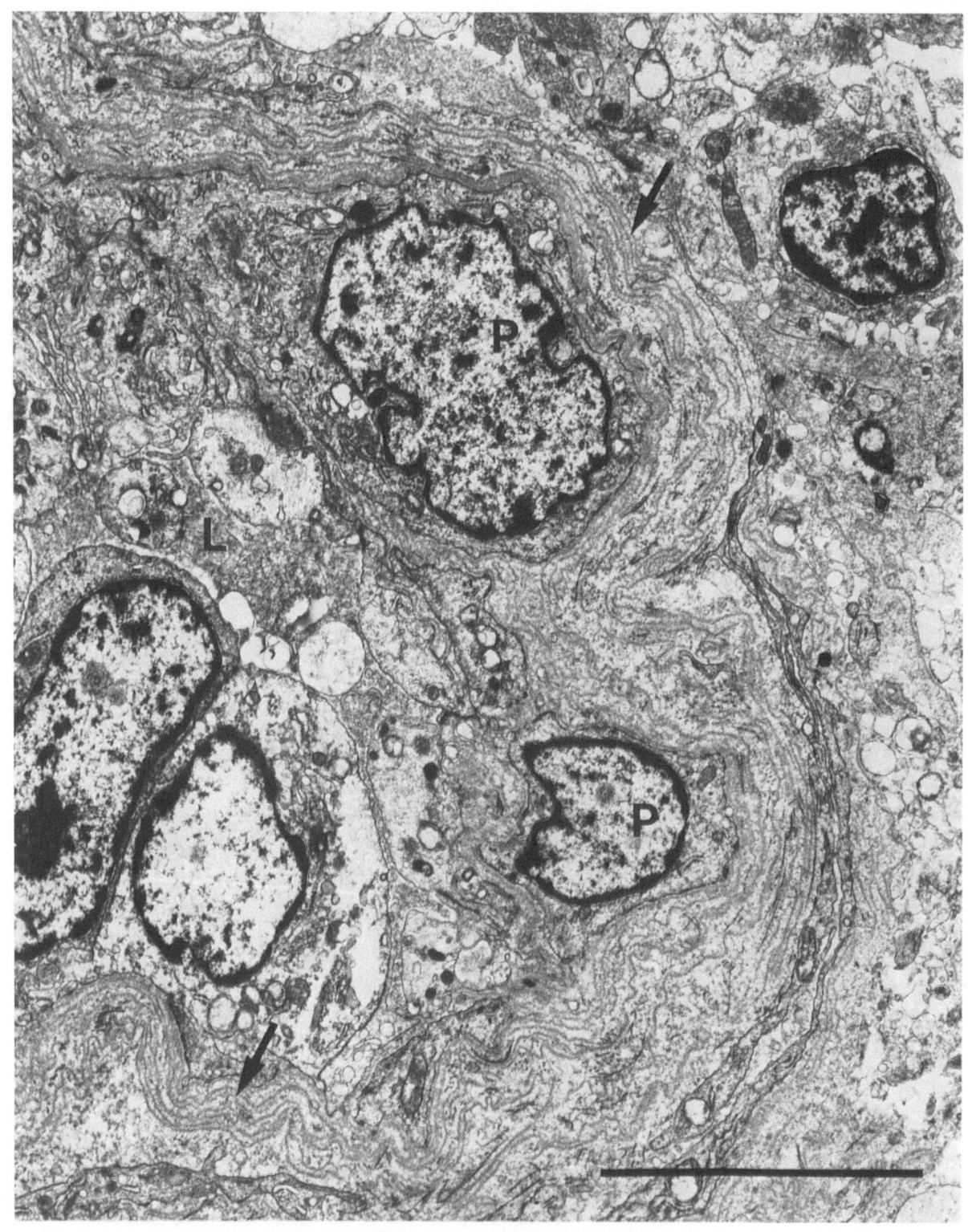

Fig. 6.3. *Malignant glioma.* Blood vessels are often hyperplastic, and their lumina (*L*) may be obliterated by swollen, proliferated endothelial cells, as seen on the *left*. In this case there is also proliferation of surrounding pericytes (*P*), which are enveloped by typical concentric reduplication of basement membrane (*arrows*). (Bar = 5 μm)

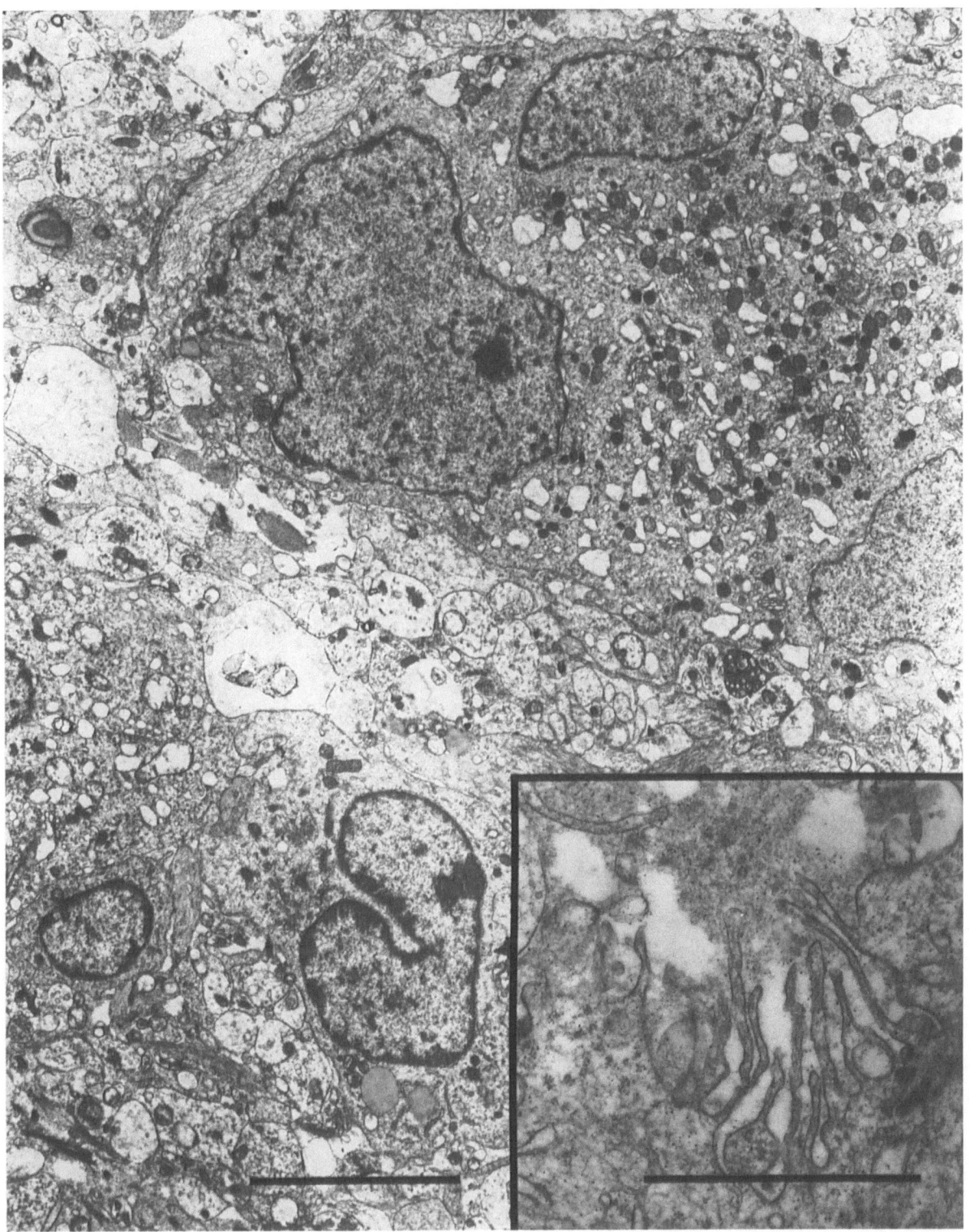

Fig. 6.4. *Glioblastoma multiforme.* These tumours usually show considerable pleomorphism and in some areas there may be numerous giant cells, like the one at the *top* of this figure, with multiple or irregularly shaped nuclei and voluminous cytoplasm. (Bar = 5 μm). *Inset*: Ruffling of tumour cell membranes, sometimes resulting in the formation of microvillous projections like these, is a characteristic feature of the more pleomorphic cells. (Bar = 2 μm)

7 Choroid Plexus Papilloma

The ultrastructural appearances of choroid plexus papillomas are very similar to those of normal choroid plexus tissue, and the many specialised features suggest that the neoplastic cells may have retained the ability to produce cerebrospinal fluid. The cells are mainly columnar in shape and are usually arranged in a papillary pattern with distinct apical–basal orientation. The outer, apical, surfaces give rise to a profusion of microvilli, and in some cases there may also be clumps of projecting cilia. These usually have the normal glial pattern of nine outer and two central tubules, but variations in structure are common. The cells are joined by regular apical junctional complexes, which include zonulae occludens and desmosomes. The closely apposed lateral surfaces of the cells lack junctions but typically show complex interdigitations. The basal surfaces are generally smooth and separated from the vascular core of the papillary fronds by a continuous basement membrane. Deep to this, the perivascular space contains collagen and fibroblastic spindle cells. The capillaries themselves have multiple, membrane-bridged fenestrations in their endothelial cell walls.

Tumour cell nuclei are rounded or polygonal and usually centrally located. The cytoplasmic matrix may show marked variation in electron density, sometimes giving the impression of separate populations of light and dark cell types. This variation in cytoplasmic density is also a feature of normal choroid plexus tissue, and may reflect the differing states of cell hydration at the time of fixation (see also Chap. 2). Cytoplasmic organelles include abundant mitochondria and parallel stacks of rough endoplasmic reticulum, often located beneath the apical surface. There may be large pools of glycogen granules, which are sometimes lost during processing, leaving irregular cytoplasmic spaces. Like cilia, glycogen is only present in normal choroid plexus tissue during embryonic life, and both these features are more often seen in tumours from infants, rather than older age groups. The cytoplasm may also contain large, lamellated or amorphous, membrane-bound inclusions, sometimes associated with bundles of irregular 6- to 15-nm filaments. The membrane-bound inclusions are probably autophagic vacuoles and, like the filamentous material, are also found in non-neoplastic choroid plexus cells, especially with advancing age.

Further Reading

Carter LP, Beggs J, Waggener JD (1972) Ultrastructure of three choroid plexus papillomas. Cancer 30: 1130–1136

Dohrman GJ, Bucy PC (1970) Human-choroid plexus: a light and electron microscopic study. J Neurosurg 33: 506–516

Wolfson WL, Brown WJ (1977) Disseminated choroid plexus papilloma. An ultrastructural study. Arch Pathol Lab Med 101: 366–368

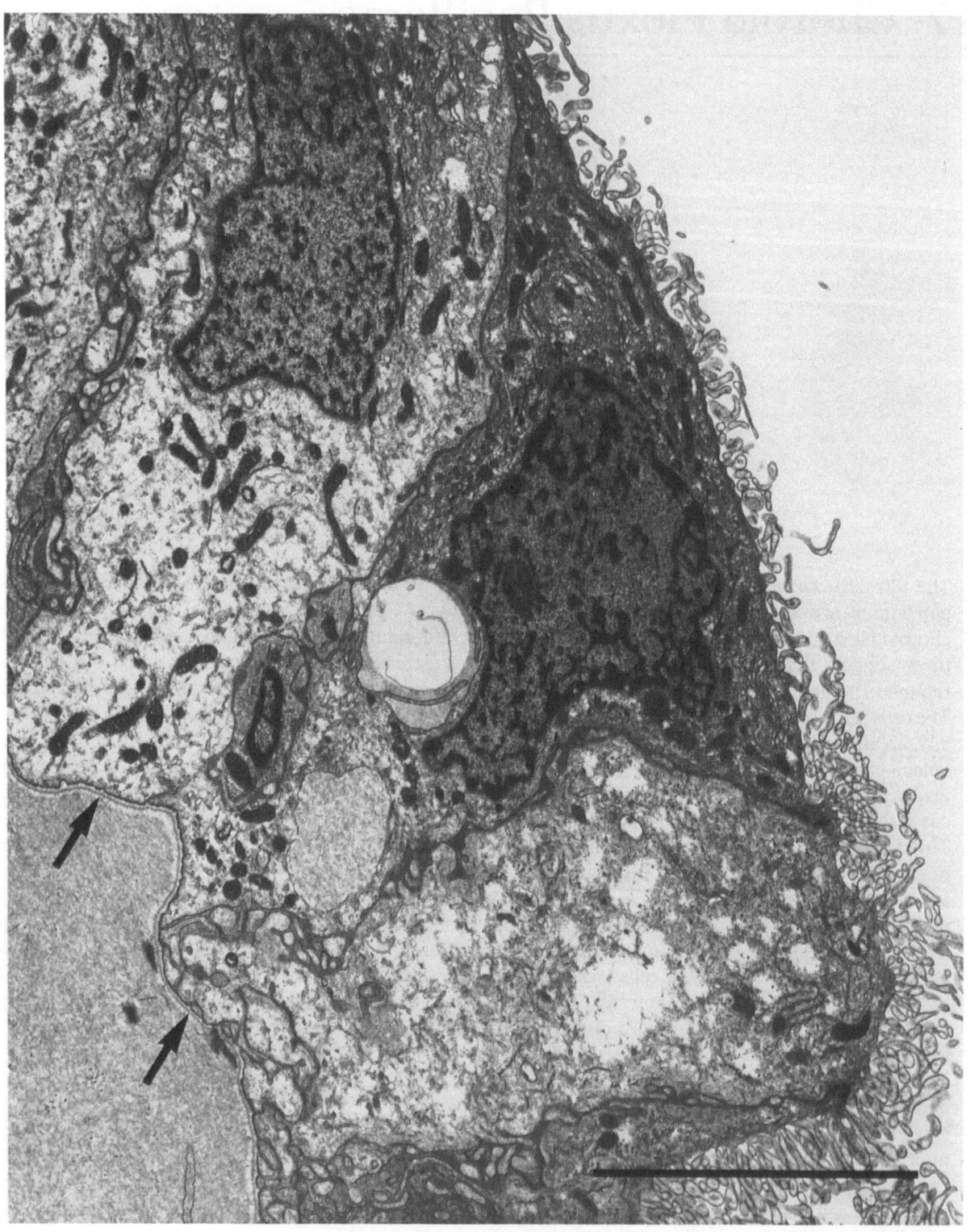

Fig. 7.1. *Choroid plexus papilloma.* The cells usually show a distinct apical–basal orientation with abundant apical microvilli, as seen on the *right*. The basal surfaces are covered by basement membrane (*arrows*). Variation in electron density of the cytoplasm may give an impression of light and dark cell types, as in this field. Glycogen present in the cells may be lost during processing, leaving irregular cytoplasmic spaces like those seen in the lowermost cell here. (Bar = 5 μm)

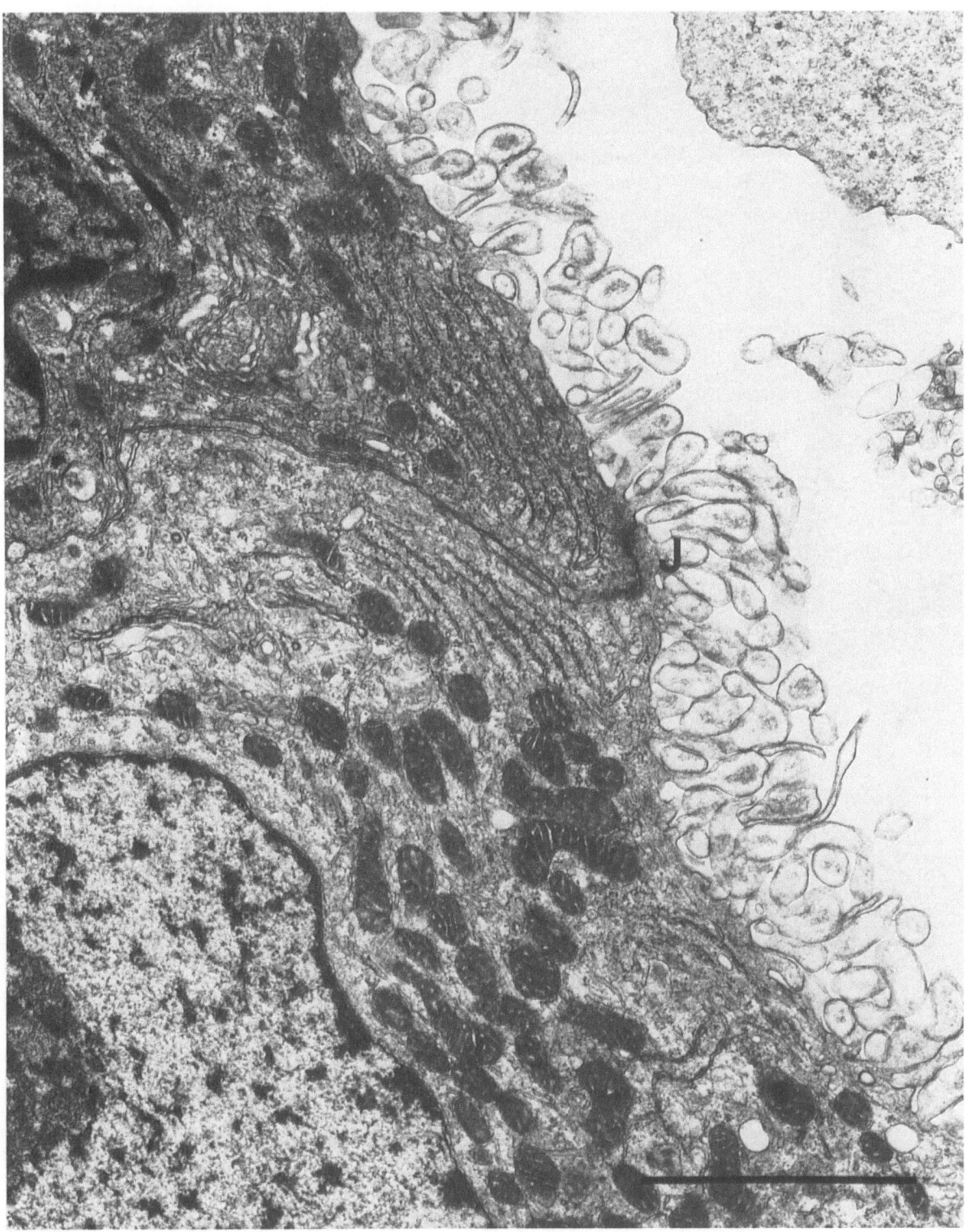

Fig. 7.2. *Choroid plexus papilloma.* The apical surfaces of adjacent cells are joined by junctional complexes (*J*), but these are not present elsewhere in the tumour. Apical microvilli, seen on the *right* of this field, are typically profuse. Both mitochondria and parallel stacks of rough endoplasmic reticulum may also be prominent features, as in the cells here. (Bar = 2 μm)

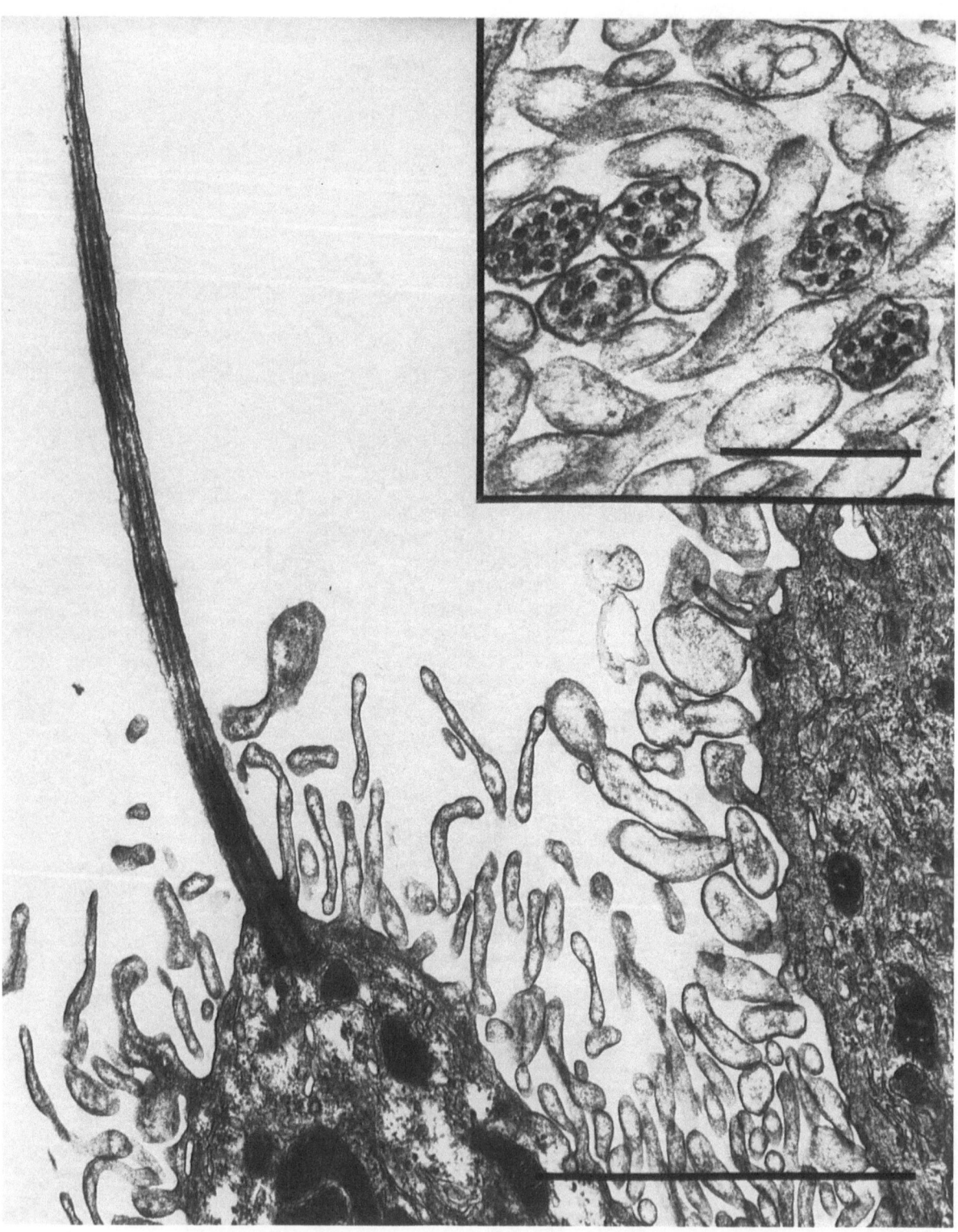

Fig. 7.3. *Choroid plexus papilloma.* Cilia may project from the apical surfaces of cells and are most commonly encountered in tumours from infants. (Bar = 2 μm). *Inset:* When present, cilia usually have the typical glial pattern of nine outer and two central tubules, but abnormal variations like those seen here are not uncommon. (Bar = 0.5 μm)

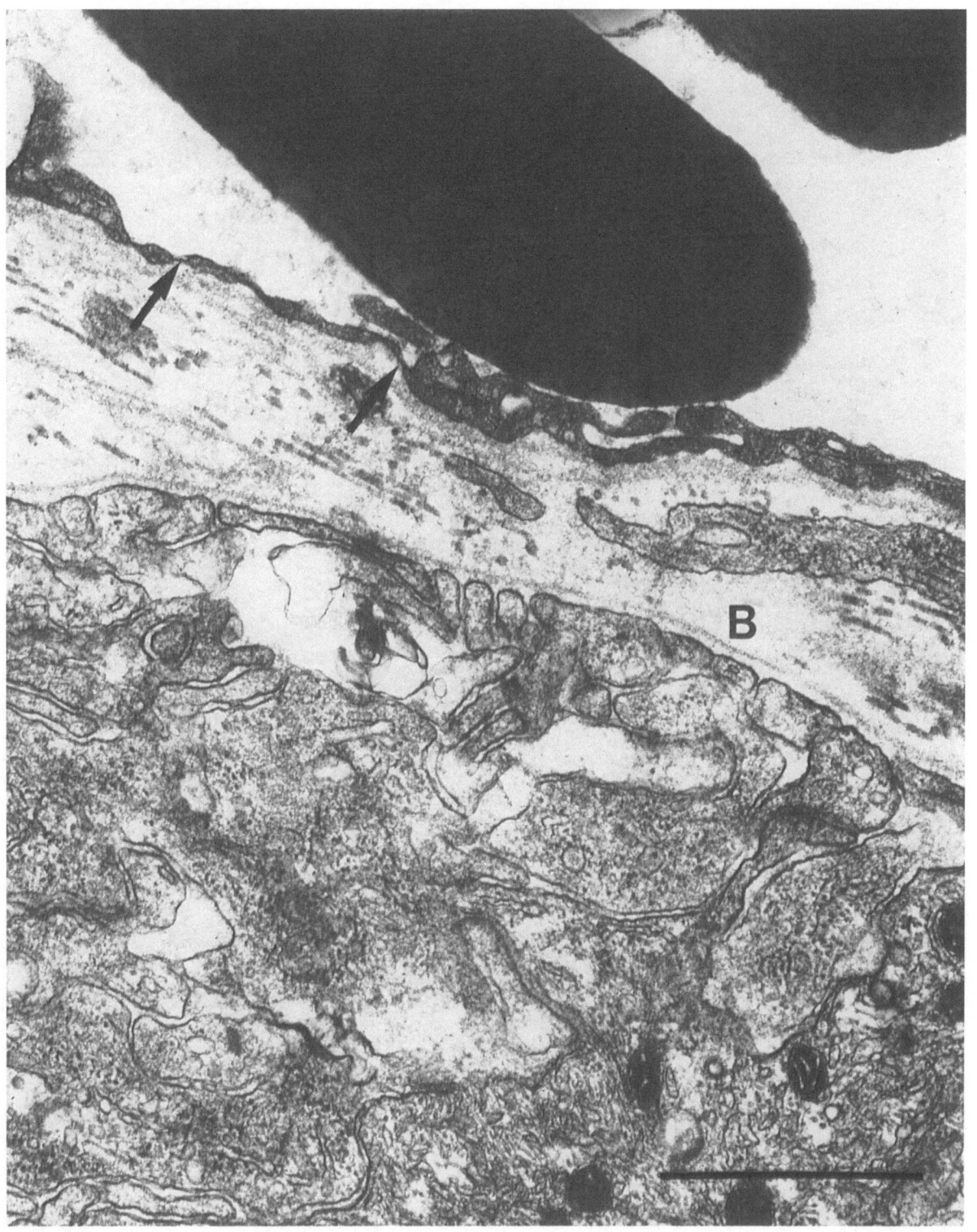

Fig. 7.4. *Choroid plexus papilloma.* The basal surfaces of tumour cells are separated from the collagen in the perivascular spaces by a continuous basement membrane (*B*). The capillary endothelium typically shows many membrane-bridged fenestrations (*arrows*). (Bar = 1 μm)

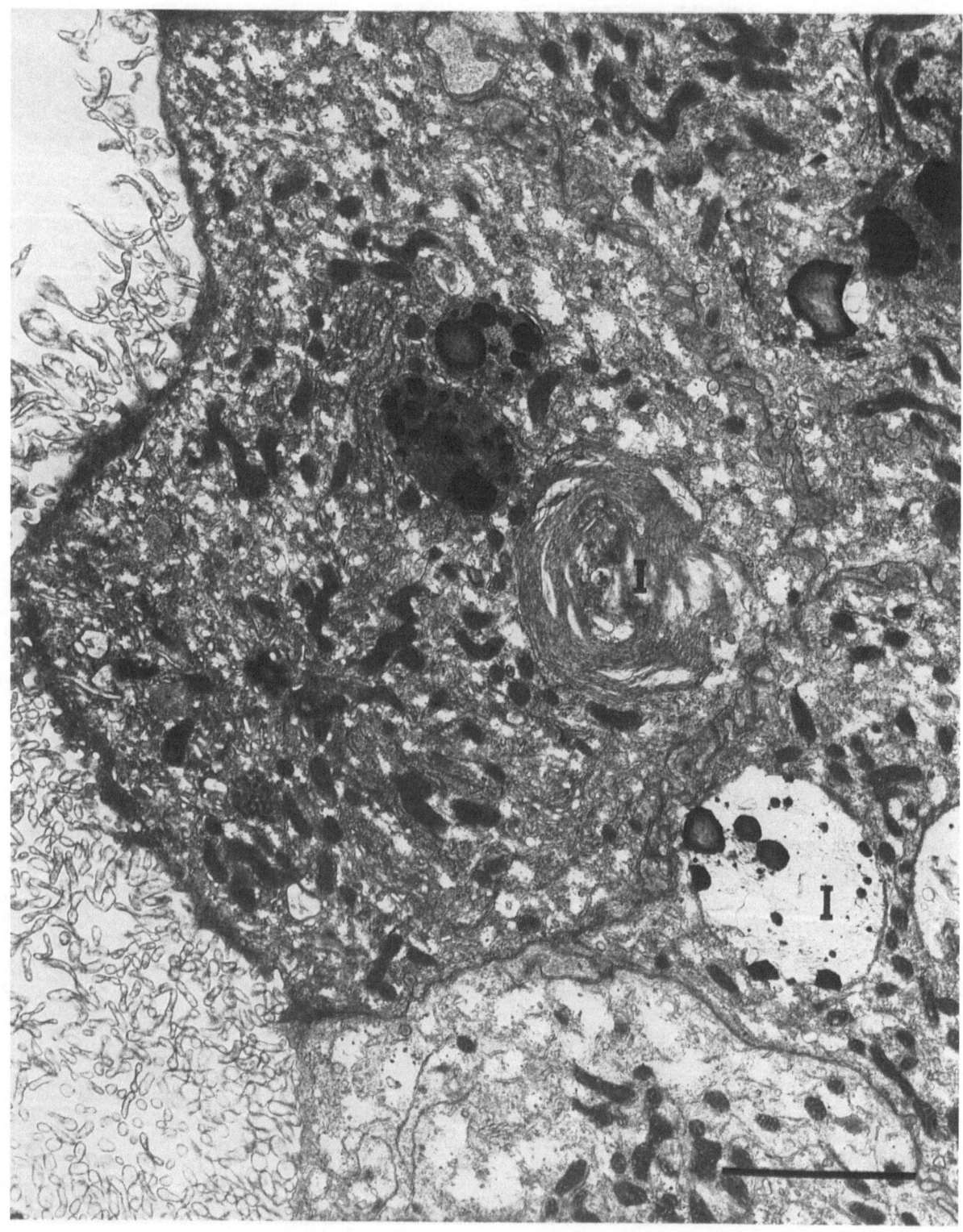

Fig. 7.5. *Choroid plexus papilloma.* Membrane-bound inclusions (*I*) may be present in the cytoplasm of many tumour cells, and contain whorled, lamellar material or osmiophilic droplets. They are probably autophagic in nature. (Bar = 2 μm)

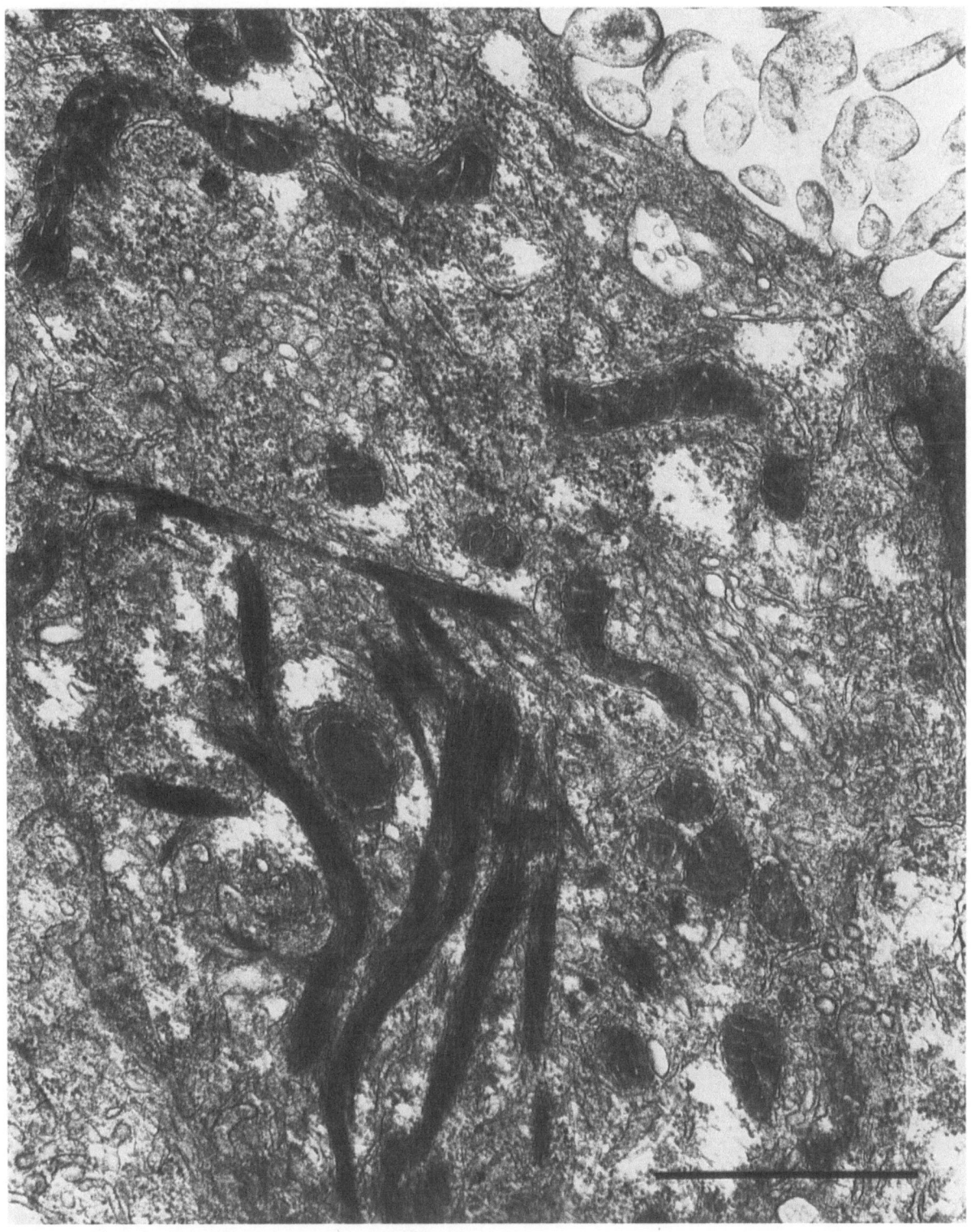

Fig. 7.6. *Choroid plexus papilloma.* Bundles of irregular, 6- to 15-nm filaments, like those present in this cell, may be associated with the membrane-bound inclusions in some instances. Both features are increasingly prominent in normal choroid plexus cells with advancing age. (Bar = 1 μm)

8 Malignant Choroid Plexus Papilloma

Malignant choroid plexus papillomas are a rare, malignant form of choroid plexus tumour, and are sometimes referred to as "choroid plexus carcinomas". These tumours are apparently distinct from benign choroid plexus papillomas, and there is no evidence that they are the result of malignant change taking place in a pre-existing benign papilloma. Using light microscopy, they can easily be mistaken for metastatic adenocarcinomas, but ultrastructurally they often retain many features typical of normal choroid plexus, and electron microscopy can thus be of great value in establishing the diagnosis.

The tumour cells generally form solid sheets with complex interdigitations, and there is loss of the prominent papillary pattern and the apical–basal orientation of cells seen in the benign papillomas. Nuclei are irregularly indented and may often be seen in the process of mitotic division. The cytoplasm usually contains abundant polyribosomes, but other organelles are sparse. Some cells, however, may contain parallel stacks of rough endoplasmic reticulum and bundles of 6- to 15-nm filaments reminiscent of those found both in benign papilloma cells and in normal choroid plexus. The large, autophagic, membrane-bound inclusions seen in benign papillomas are not usually a feature of these malignant tumours.

In some areas, tumour cells may form a border with large areas of extracellular space, and occasionally such cells are joined by apical junctional complexes. Unlike the complexes in benign choroid plexus papillomas, however, these are inconstant and poorly formed, often consisting only of isolated zonulae adherentes. Microvilli may also be present on the free surfaces of such cells, although in many cases they are stunted and poorly formed, or entirely absent. Cilia are extremely rare, and tend to be buried within cell bodies, rather than projecting from the surface. As in the benign tumours, a continuous basement membrane separates the tumour cells from collagen in the perivascular spaces. Capillary endothelial fenestrations may also be found, but they are much less numerous than in the vessels of benign papillomas or normal choroid plexus tissue.

Further Reading

Boesel CP, Suhan JP (1979) A pigmented choroid plexus carcinoma: histochemical and ultrastructural studies. J Neuropathol Exp Neurol 38: 177–186

Gullotta F, DeMelo AS, (1979) Carcinomas and malignant papillomas of the choroid plexus. Neurochir (Stuttg) 22: 1–9

Moss TH (1983) Electron microscopic observations on malignant choroid plexus papilloma. Neuropathol Appl Neurobiol 9: 225–235

Nakashima N, Goto K, Takeuchi J (1982) Papillary carcinoma of choroid plexus. Light and electron microscopic study. Virchows Arch [A] 395: 303–318

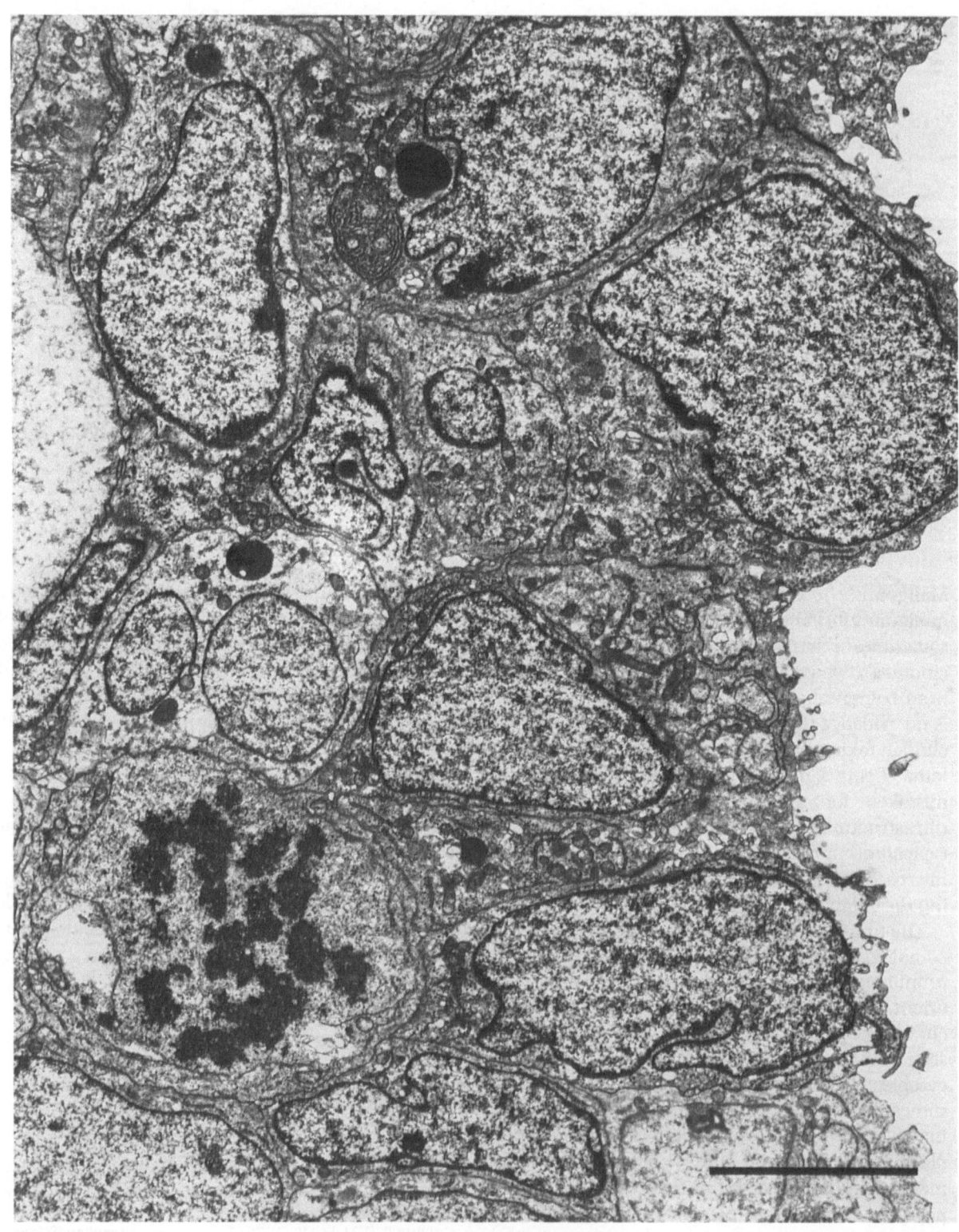

Fig. 8.1. *Malignant choroid plexus papilloma.* In most areas the cells form solid sheets, usually without obvious apical–basal orientation. Nuclei are pleomorphic and there are frequent mitotic figures, like that at the *bottom left*. In some areas the cells may border large extracellular spaces, as on the *right*, but the exposed cell surfaces often lack well-formed microvillous processes. (Bar = 5 μm) (Moss 1983)

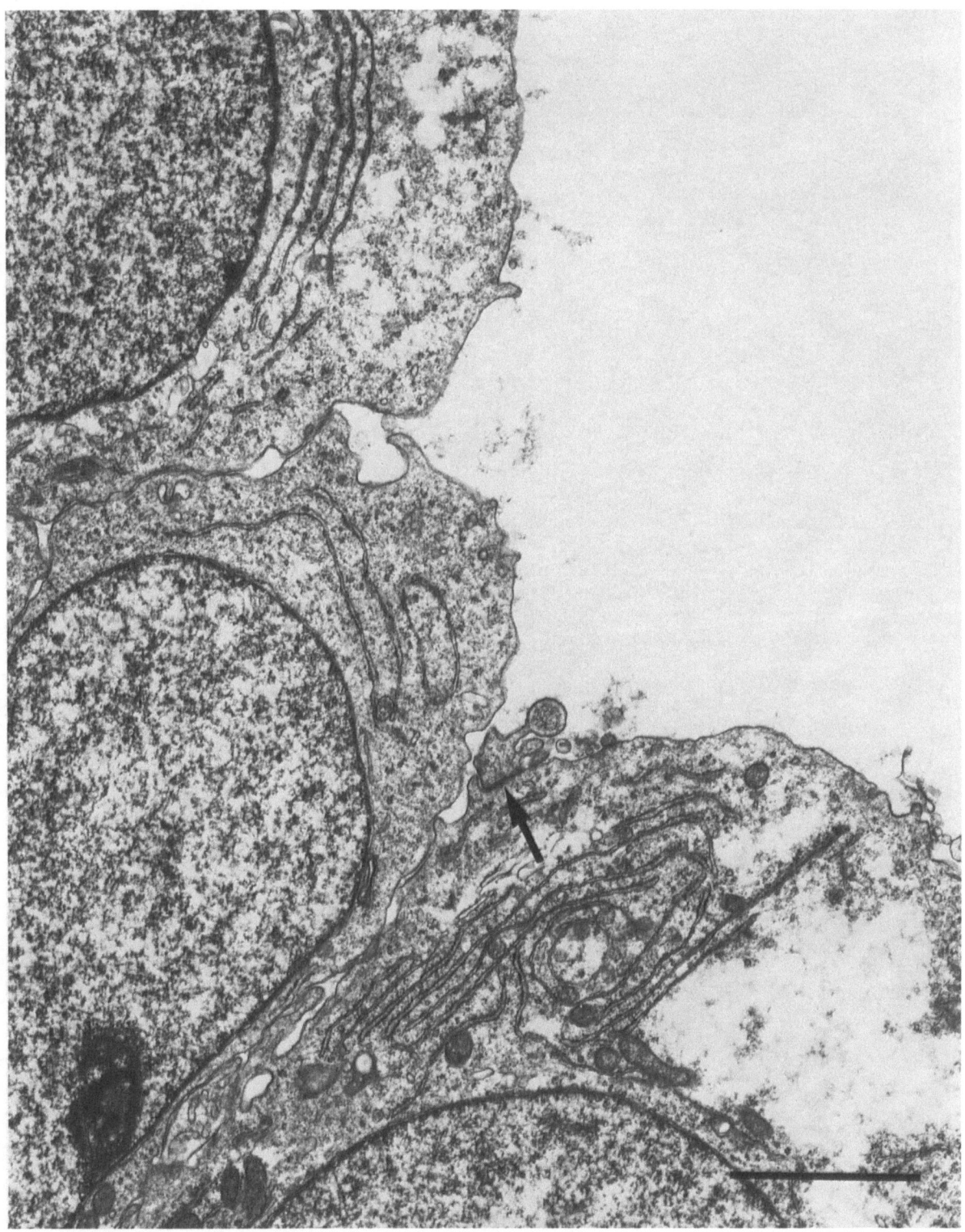

Fig. 8.2. *Malignant choroid plexus papilloma.* The cell cytoplasm is largely filled by polyribosomes in most instances, but there may also be parallel stacks of rough endoplasmic reticulum, as in the cells shown here. Cells bordering extracellular space, like these, often lack microvilli and apical junctional complexes, but occasional zonulae adherentes junctions may be present near the free surfaces of adjacent cells (*arrow*). (Bar = 2 μm) (Moss 1983)

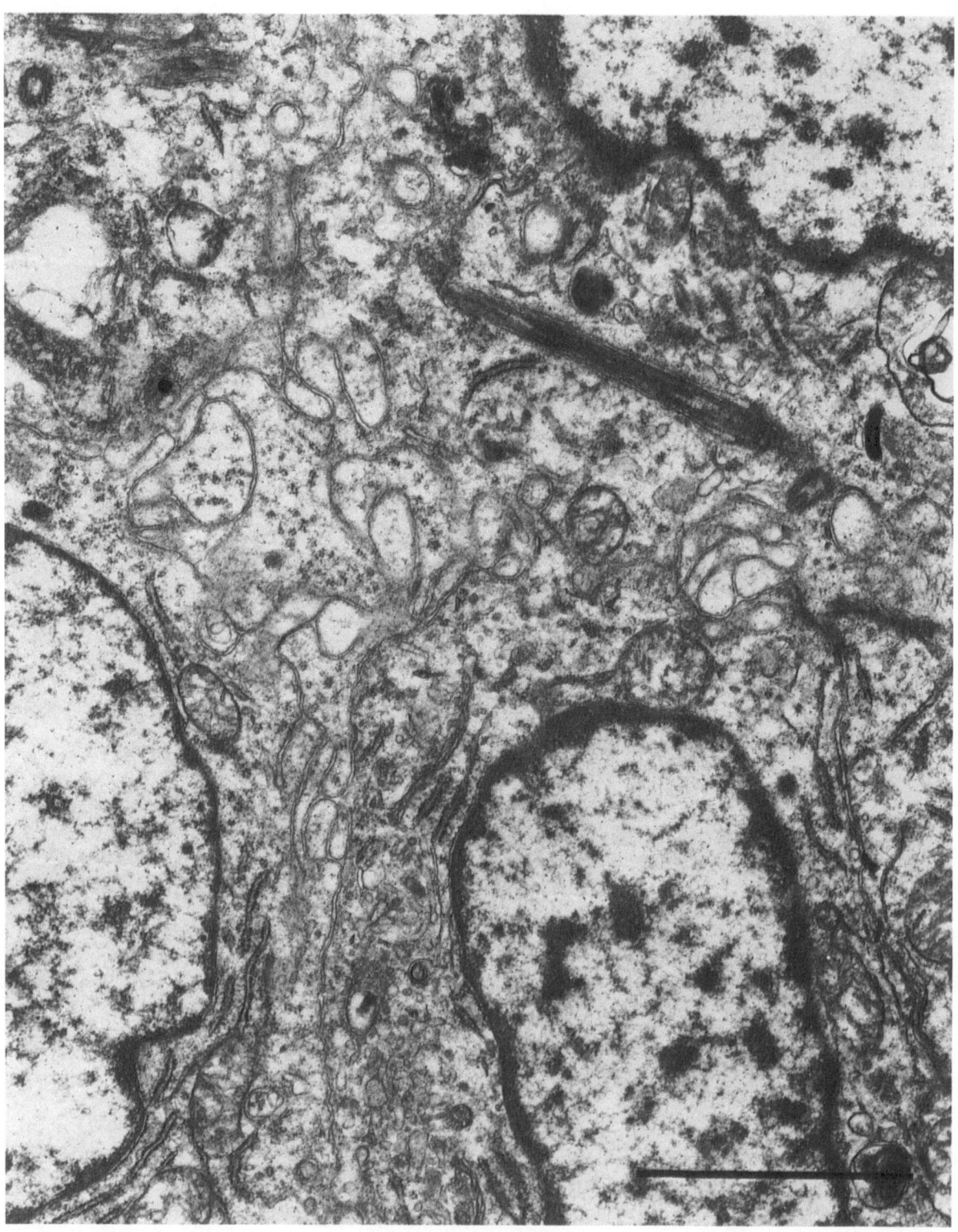

Fig. 8.3. *Malignant choroid plexus papilloma*. The cells are usually irregularly but tightly packed together and may show complex interdigitations, as in the *centre* of this field. Cilia are extremely rare, and like the one seen towards the *top* of this figure, they tend to be buried within cell bodies. (Bar = 2 μm) (Moss 1983)

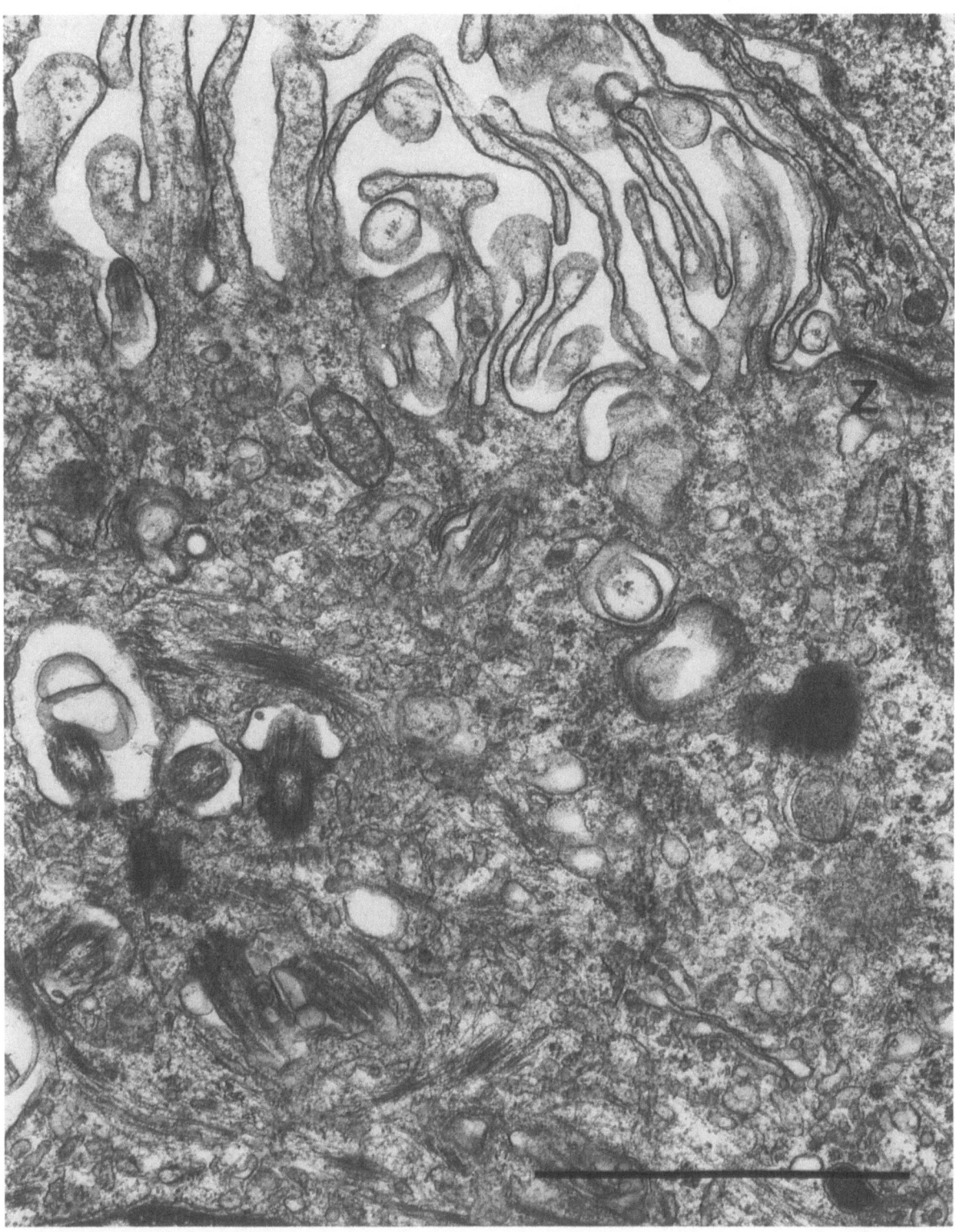

Fig. 8.4. *Malignant choroid plexus papilloma.* In better differentiated areas, cells bordering extracellular space may form microvilli, as seen at the *top* of this figure. An apical zonula adherentes junction is also present in this instance (Z). The basal bodies and bundles of filamentous material present on the *left* are similar to those found in benign choroid plexus papillomas. (Bar = 2 μm) (Moss 1983)

9 Primary Pineal Tumours

Pineocytomas and pineoblastomas have many features in common at ultrastructural level, and appear to be represent two ends of a spectrum of tumours which includes many intermediate forms.

Typical pineocytomas reproduce many features of the normal human pineal gland, including ganglionic differentiation and a characteristic arrangement of perivascular processes. They are fundamentally neuroblastic tumours and also share many ultrastructural characteristics with primary cerebral neuroblastomas, from which they differ largely by virtue of their specialised site in the pineal gland. Cell bodies are typically arranged in clumps which are separated by numerous, fine, interlacing processes. Nuclei are rounded, with finely granular chromatin and rather poorly defined nucleoli. The electron-lucent perinuclear cytoplasm is usually abundant and contains varied organelles, including neurosecretory dense-core vesicles. These vesicles have a distinctive appearance, with an electron-lucent halo separating the rounded, dense core from an outer membrane. They are often larger than those seen in neuroblastomas, and may have an external diameter of up to 300 nm. The interlacing cell processes are electron lucent and usually resemble neuritic processes. They contain longitudinally orientated 20-nm microtubules, dense-core vesicles and large numbers of smaller, 40- to 60-nm diameter synaptic vesicles. The latter are frequently aggregated next to desmosome-like membrane thickenings, producing structures resembling synaptic complexes. Around blood vessels, cell processes are closely applied to the outer basement membrane and often have characteristic, club-shaped terminal expansions. Scattered astrocytic processes filled with 6- to 9-nm glial filaments are usually interspersed with the neuritic-type processes and may be numerous in some areas. They have been interpreted as evidence of divergent, astrocytic tumour differentiation, but may simply be reactive, pre-existing glial elements of the pineal gland.

Towards the pineoblastic end of the spectrum, tumours often lack many of the specialised ganglionic features of pineocytomas, and show a more primitive ultrastructural appearance. The cell bodies tend to be more pleomorphic and densely packed together, with fewer interlacing processes. Nuclei are larger, irregularly indented and often have prominent nucleoli. Perinuclear cytoplasm is usually scanty and contains few organelles other than polyribosomes. In some instances, however, these more primitive tumours may show evidence of photoreceptor differentiation, which is similar to that found in retinoblastomas and apparently recapitulates the photoreceptor role of the pineal gland in lower order animals. A variety of specialised organelles may be present in such rare cases, including vesicle-crowned lamellae (see Chap. 10), microtubular sheaves, annulate lamellae and bulbous, neuronal-type cilia like those seen in the fleurettes of retinoblastic rosettes.

Further Reading

Hassoun J, Gambarelli D, Peragut JC, Toga M (1983) Specific ultrastructural markers of human pinealomas. Acta Neuropathol 62: 31–40

Herrick MK, Rubinstein LJ (1979) The cytological differentiating potential of pineal parenchymal neoplasms (true pinealomas). A clinicopathological study of 28 tumours. Brain 102: 289–320

Kline KT, Damjanor I, Katz SM, Schmidek H (1979) Pineoblastomas: an electron microscopic study. Cancer 44: 1692–1699

Markesberry WR, Haugh RM, Young AB (1981) Ultrastructure of pineal parenchymal neoplasms. Acta Neuropathol 55: 143–149

Nielson SL, Wilson BB (1975) Ultrastructure of a 'pineocytoma'. J Neuropathol Exp Neurol 34: 148–158

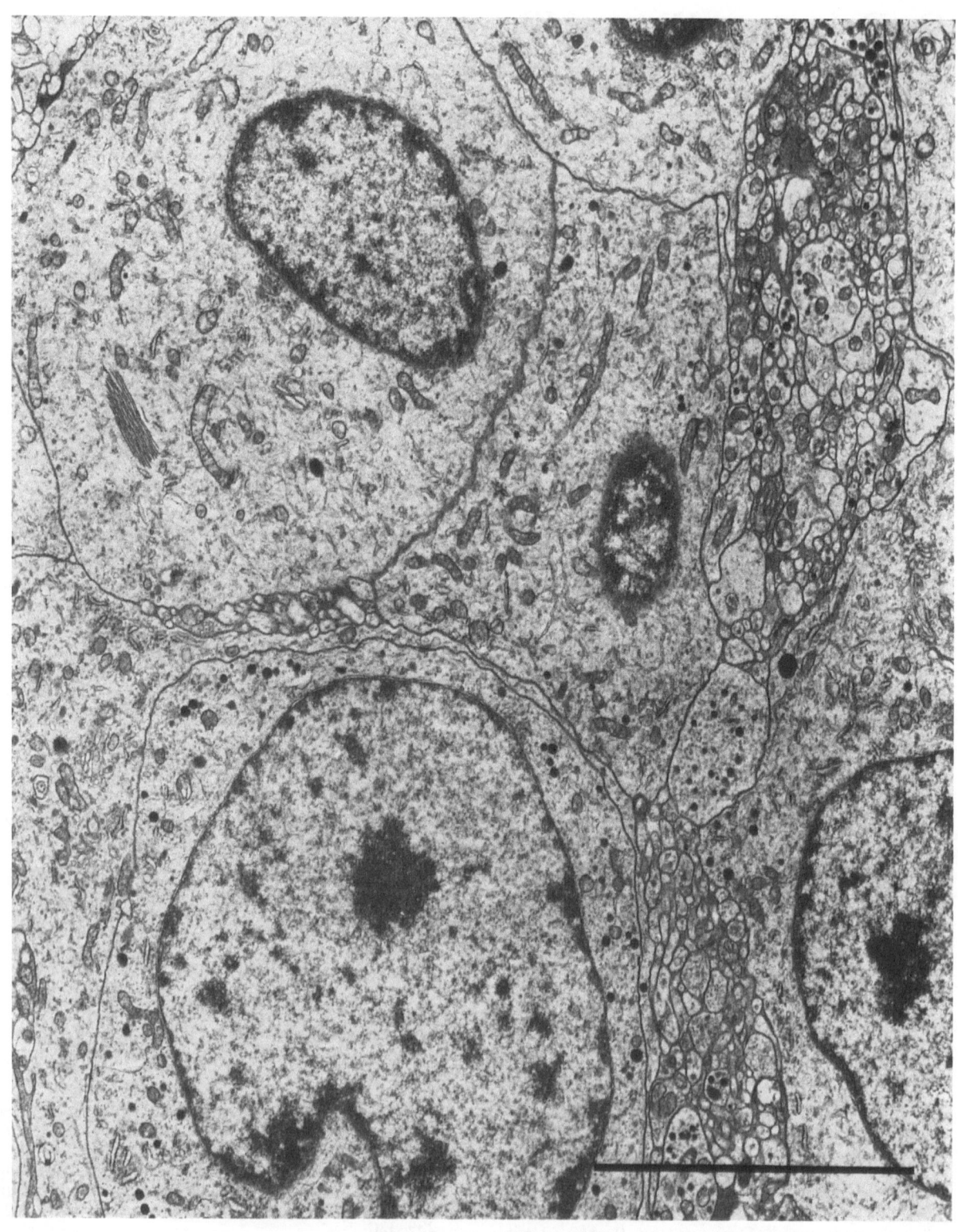

Fig. 9.1. *Pineocytoma.* Typical tumour cells have rounded nuclei with finely granular chromatin, and abundant, electron-lucent perinuclear cytoplasm. They are usually arranged in groups which are separated by fine interlacing processes, like those seen on the *right*. Dense-core vesicles are present in both cells and processes, and are visible as black dots at this magnification. (Bar = 5 μm)

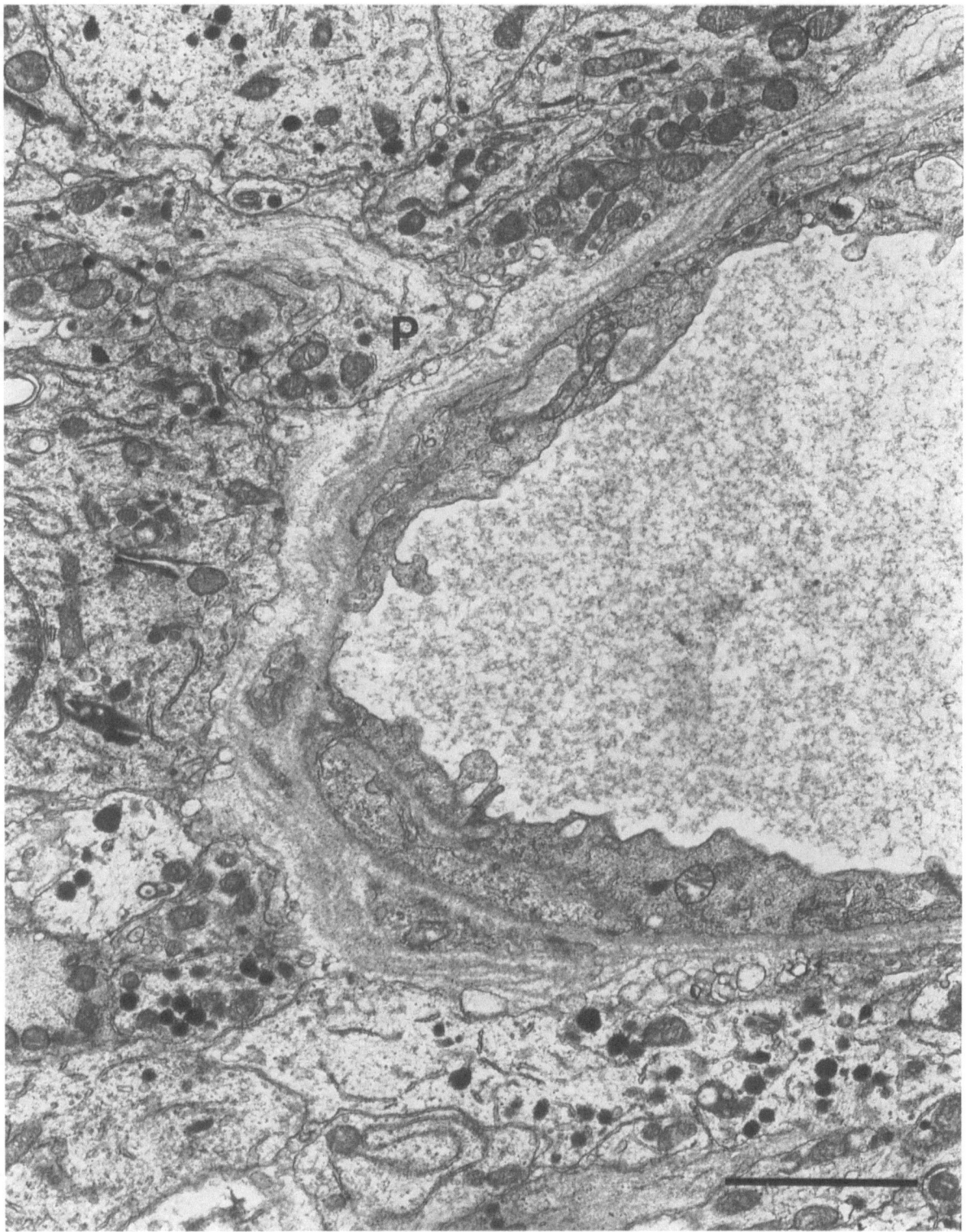

Fig. 9.2. *Pineocytoma.* Around blood vessels, the architecture is often reminiscent of that in the normal pineal gland. Tumour cell processes containing dense-core vesicles are closely applied to the outer vascular basement membrane, and frequently have club-shaped endings, like that marked *P*. (Bar = 2 μm)

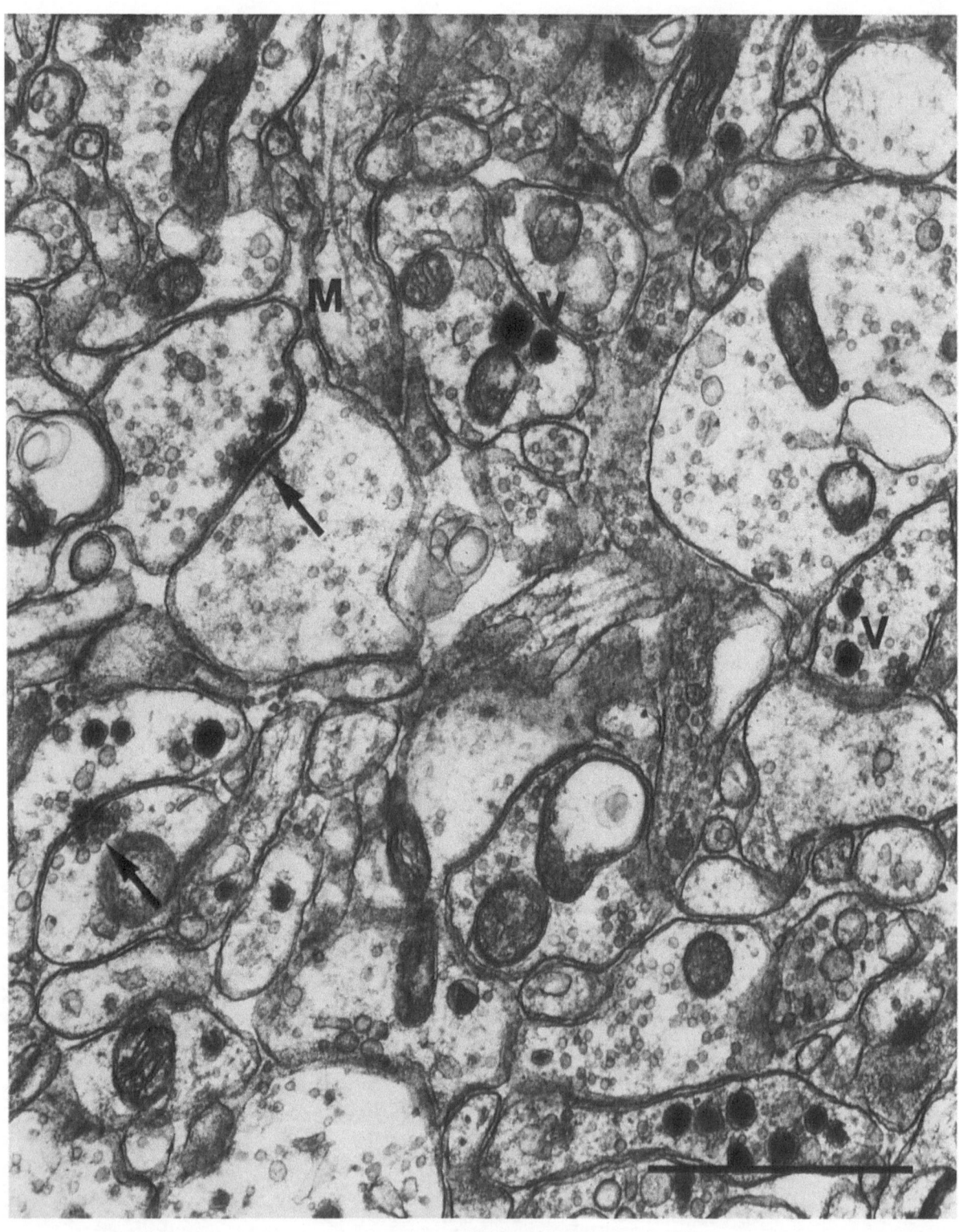

Fig. 9.3. *Pineocytoma*. The tumour cell processes often resemble neurites, as in this figure, and contain 20-nm microtubules (*M*), dense-core vesicles (*V*) and smaller 40- to 60-nm diameter synaptic vesicles. The latter are sometimes aggregated next to desmosome-like membrane thickenings to form synaptic structures (*arrows*). The larger, dense-core vesicles are up to 300 nm in diameter and have a characteristic clear halo between the dense granule and the outer membrane. (Bar = 1 μm)

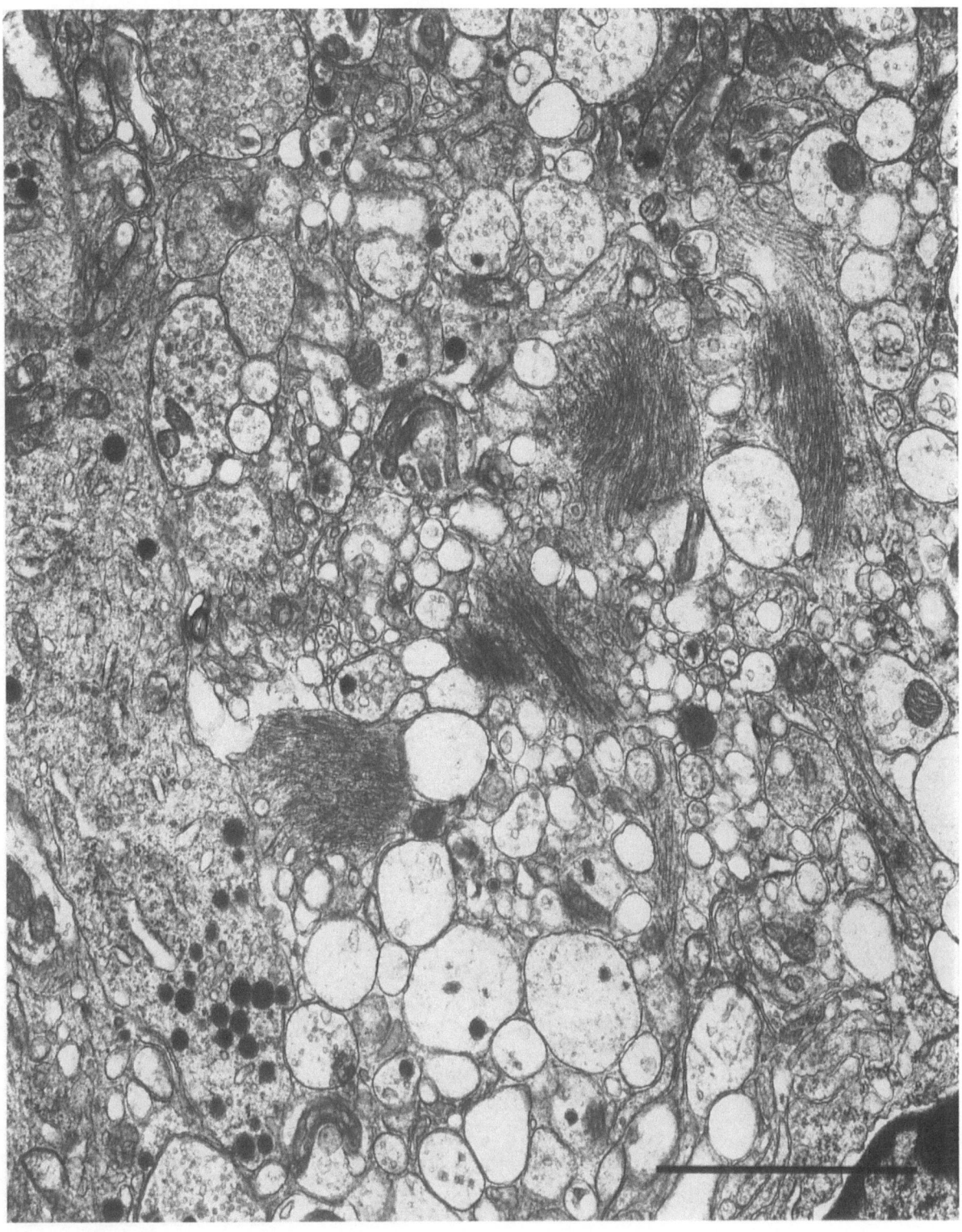

Fig. 9.4. *Pineocytoma.* Astrocytic processes filled with 6- to 9-nm glial filaments are often a prominent feature of these tumours, as in the field shown here. They probably represent reactive, pre-existing glial elements of the pineal gland. (Bar = 1 μm)

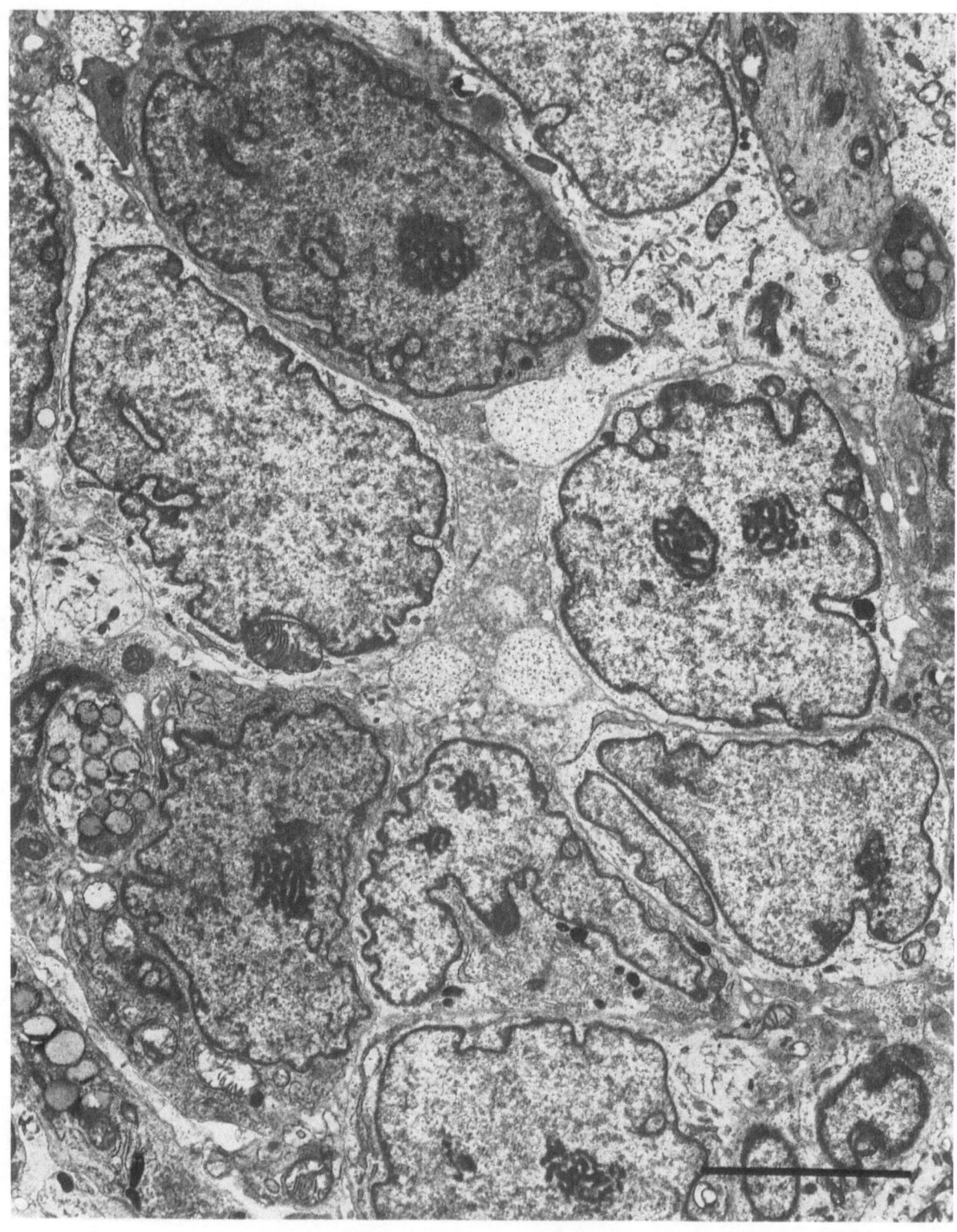

Fig. 9.5. *Pineoblastoma.* These tumours tend to have a more primitive appearance, as in the example illustrated here. The tumour cell nuclei are large and irregular with prominent nucleoli, and the scanty perinuclear cytoplasm contains mainly polyribosomes. In contrast to pineocytomas, the cells usually show little tendency to form interlacing, neuritic-type processes. (Bar = 5 μm)

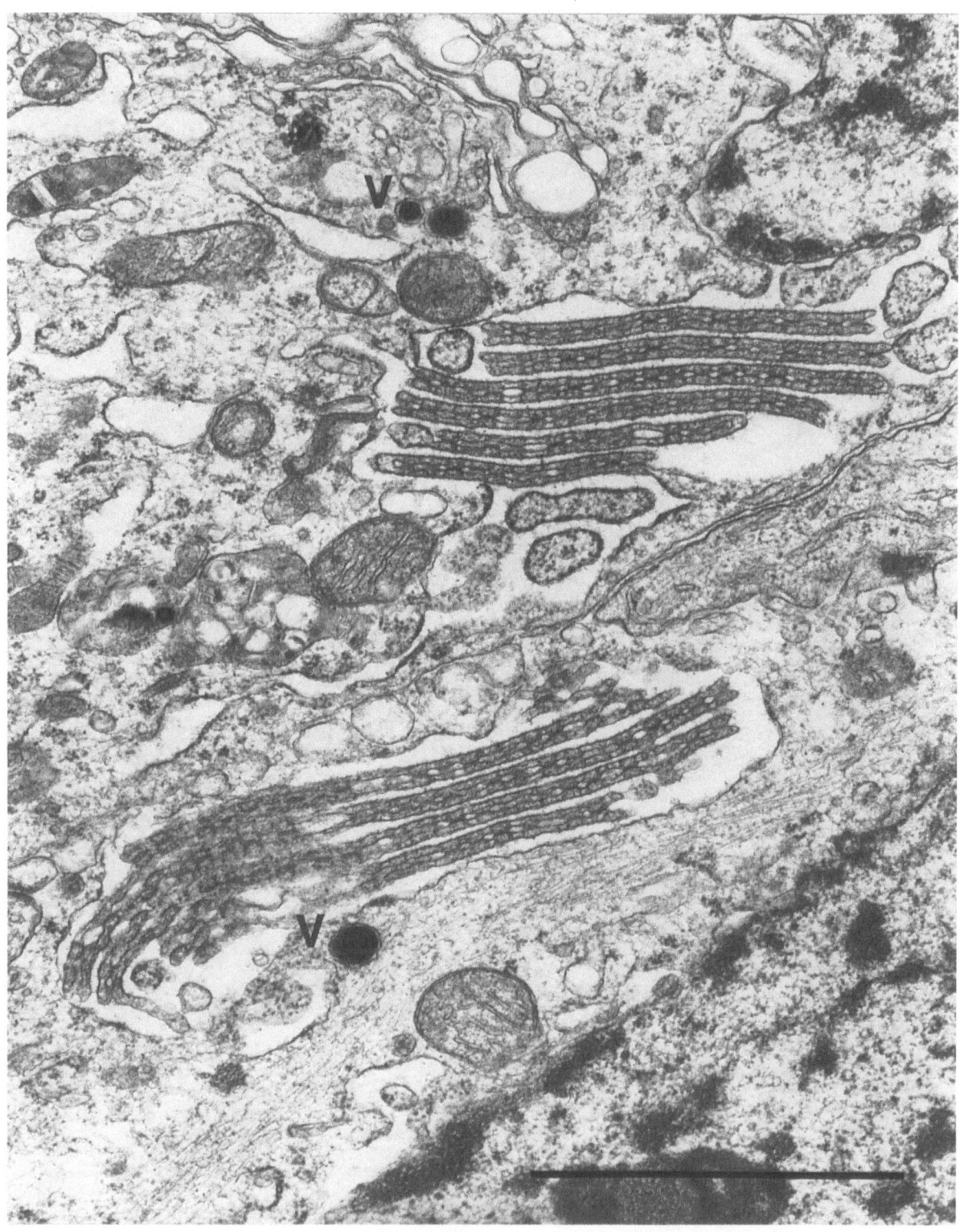

Fig. 9.6. *Pineoblastoma.* The tumour cells usually contain scattered dense-core vesicles (*V*), although they may be hard to find in poorly differentiated cases. In this case, some of the cells also contained these unusually well-formed, paracrystalline annulate lamellae, a feature more typically associated with testicular seminomas and retinoblastomas. (Bar = 2 μm)

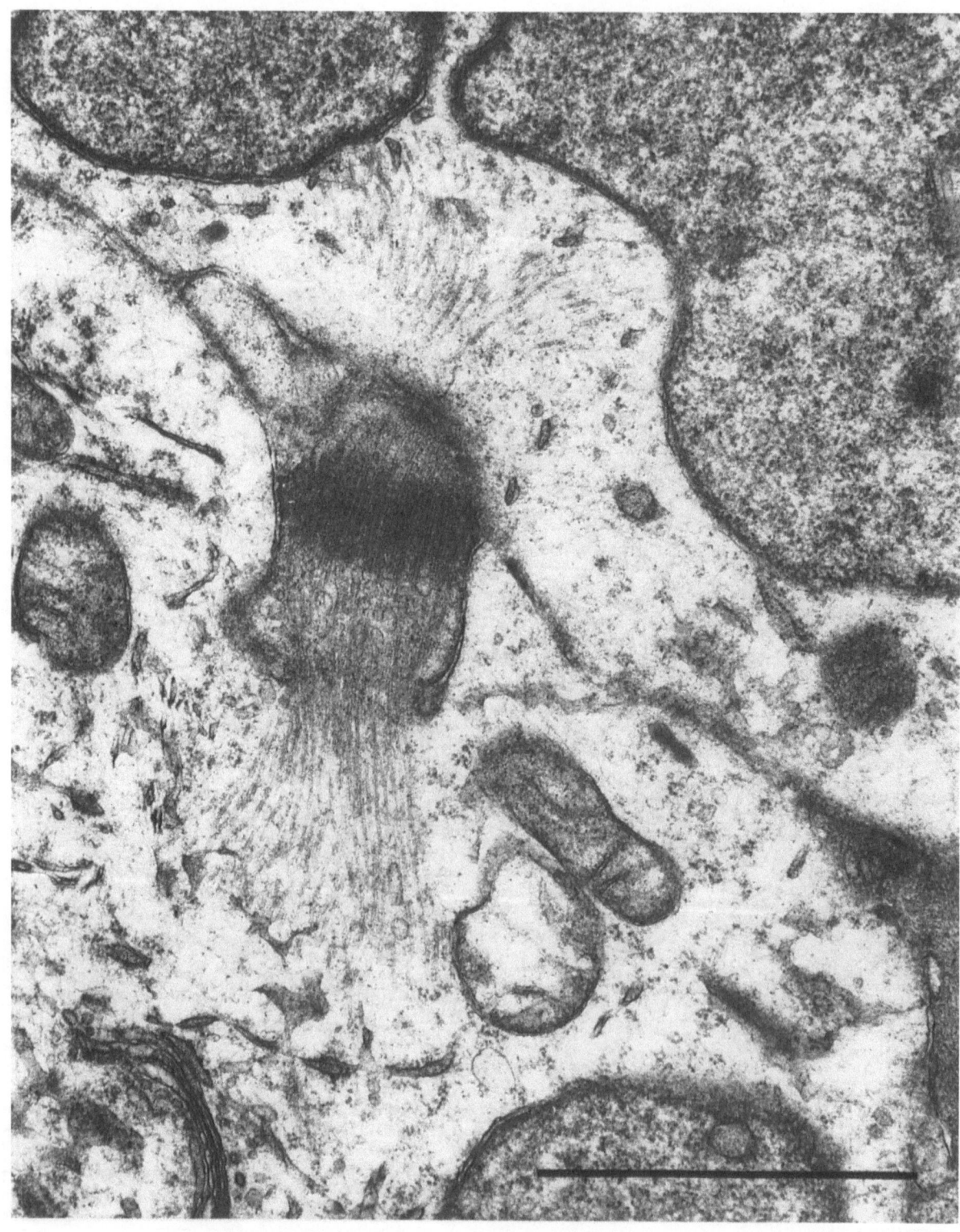

Fig. 9.7. *Pineoblastoma with evidence of photoreceptor differentiation.* This unusual tumour contained structures resembling microtubular sheaves, like the one illustrated here. These are similar to the microtubular sheaves found in retinoblastomas, but much broader, with larger numbers of 20-nm microtubules aggregated together. (Bar = 2 μm)

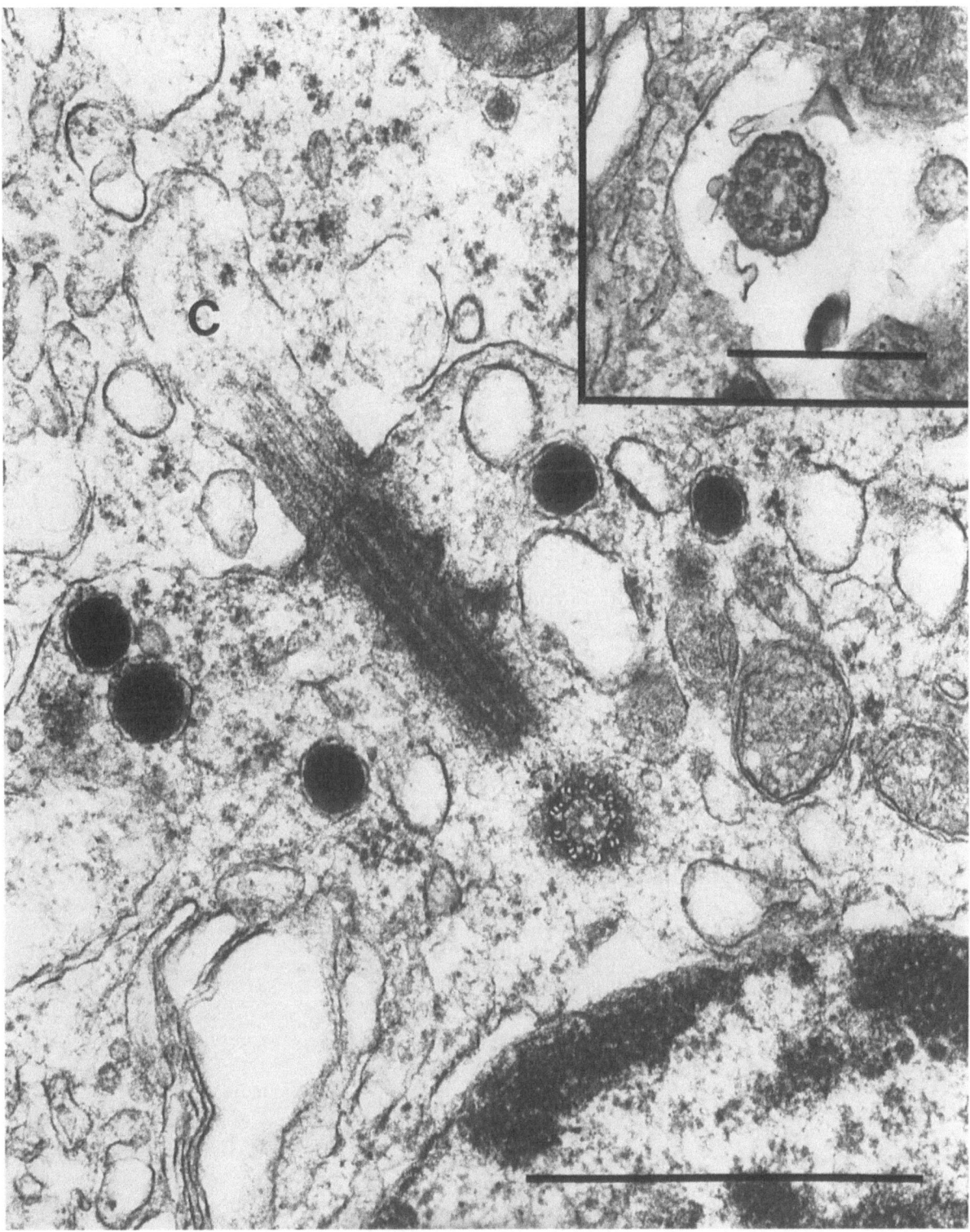

Fig. 9.8. *Pineoblastoma with evidence of photoreceptor differentiation.* This tumour contained bulb-ended cilia (*C*), similar to those found in the fleurettes of retinoblastic rosettes. Typical dense-core vesicles are also present in this field, with clearly visible electron-lucent halos separating the central granules from the outer membranes. (Bar = 1 μm) *Inset*: The cilia are of neuronal type, with nine outer paired tubules but no central ones, as demonstrated here in cross-section. (Bar = 0.5 μm)

10 Medulloblastoma

Medulloblastomas are primitive neuroectodermal tumours which probably originate from persistent external granule layer neuroblasts of the foetal cerebellum. At ultrastructural level, the tumour cells appear rounded or angular and form a closely packed mosaic with little intervening extracellular space. Adjacent cells often deeply indent each other, producing a characteristic moulding or distortion of their cytoplasm and nuclei. The nuclei themselves are deeply invaginated, and typically show multiple lobulation. Nuclear chromatin is finely granular and there may be an occasional, peripherally located nucleolus. There is usually only a thin rim of perinuclear cytoplasm, which contains poly-ribosomes but few other organelles. Junction-like membrane densities may be present between cells, but are inconstant and poorly formed. In many cases the tumour cells form thin, electron-lucent processes, which contain 20-nm microtubules and may resemble those found in neuroblastic tumours. Homer-Wright rosettes are formed from an outer circle of cell bodies, usually lacking specialised features, and have a solid, central area of interlacing cell processes. Blood vessels are unremarkable, with an intact outer basement membrane and non-fenestrated endothelial cells. Phagocytic cells, containing numerous cytoplasmic lipid droplets, may be numerous in some cases. The processes and cell bodies of typical fibrillary astrocytes may also intersperse with tumour cells, and probably represent pre-existing, reactive, glial cells of the infiltrated cerebellum.

Although the majority of these tumours appear entirely primitive using light microscopy, some electron microscopic evidence of both glial and neuroblastic differentiation can be found in many cases, and in rare examples may be very prominent. Occasional tumour cells with otherwise typical ultrastructural morphology may contain bundles of 6- to 9-nm filaments, indicating glial differentiation. In extreme cases, usually detectable by light microscopy, there may be numerous gemistocyte-like tumour cells entirely filled with glial filaments. Many largely primitive tumours may also contain unipolar cells, with prominent nucleoli and tapering terminal processes suggesting neuroblastic differentiation. In rare cases, again usually apparent by light microscopy, there may be frank ganglionic differentiation with synapses, dense-core vesicles and other neuroblastic organelles such as synaptic (or "vesicle-crowned") lamellae. Both glial and ganglionic features may be present within the same tumour, suggesting that all medulloblastomas may have a bipotential differentiating capacity. In support of this concept, similar divergent differentiation has also been demonstrated following experimental tissue culture of initially primitive medulloblastoma cells.

Further Reading

Cummins MB, Cravioto HM, Epstein F, Ransohoff J (1980) Medulloblastoma: an ultrastructural study—evidence for astrocytic and neuronal differentiation. Neurosurgery 6: 398–411

Matakas F, Cervós-Navarro J, Gullota F (1976) The ultra-structure of medulloblastoma. Acta Neuropathol 16: 271–284

Moss TH (1983) Evidence for differentiation in medulloblastomas appearing primitive on light microscopy: an ultrastructural study. Histopathology 7: 919–930

Roy S (1977) An ultrastructural study of medulloblastoma. Neurol India 25: 226–229

Rubinstein LJ, Herman MM, Hanberry JW (1974) The relationship between differentiating medulloblastoma and de-differentiating diffuse cerebellar astrocytoma. Cancer 33: 675–690

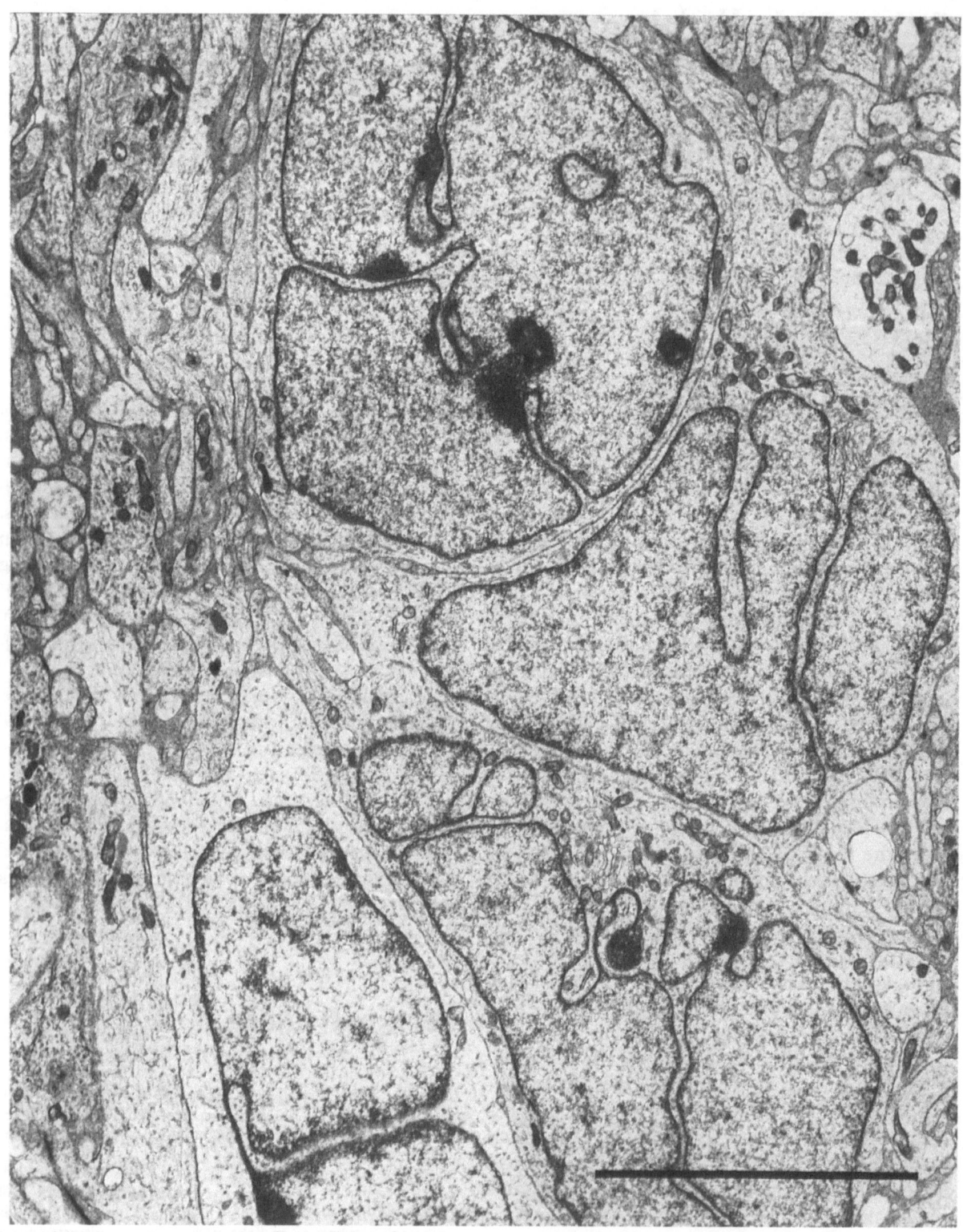

Fig. 10.1. *Medulloblastoma.* Tumour cell nuclei are large and frequently show the characteristic lobulation seen here. There is usually only a scanty rim of perinuclear cytoplasm containing mainly polyribosomes, but fine cell processes may also be present, like those seen on the *left*. As with the upper two cells here, the bodies of adjacent tumour cells often indent each other, producing a typical moulding of their cytoplasm and nuclei. (Bar = 5 μm)

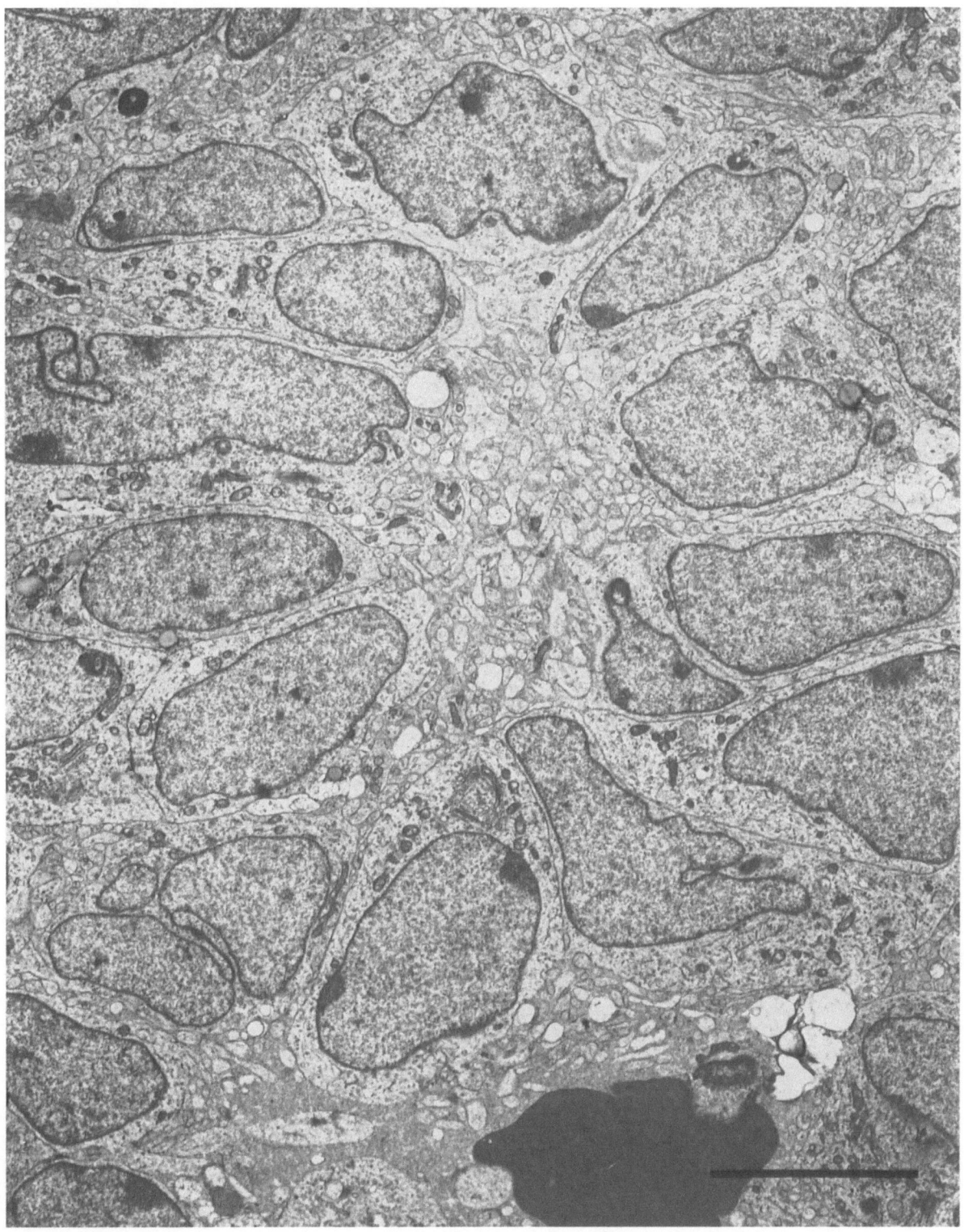

Fig. 10.2. *Medulloblastoma*. Homer-Wright rosettes, such as the one illustrated, are formed by an outer circle of tumour cell bodies which usually lack specialised features. The solid central area is filled by interlacing tumour cell processes. (Bar = 5 μm) (Moss 1983)

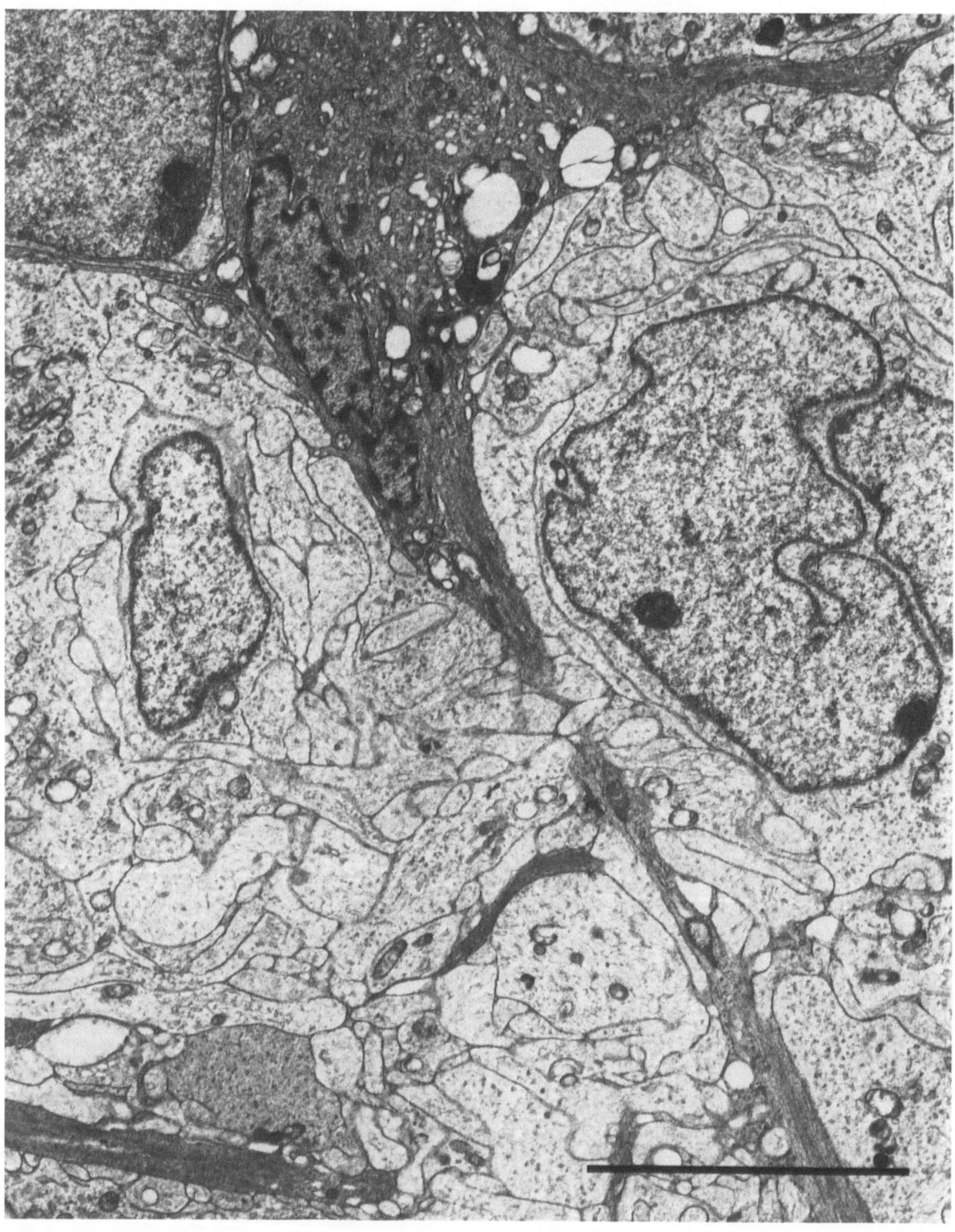

Fig. 10.3. *Medulloblastoma.* Tumour cells and interlacing processes may be interspersed with typical, filament-containing, fibrillary astrocytes, like the one at the *top* of this figure. These cells probably represent reactive glial elements of the infiltrated nervous tissue. (Bar = 5 μm)

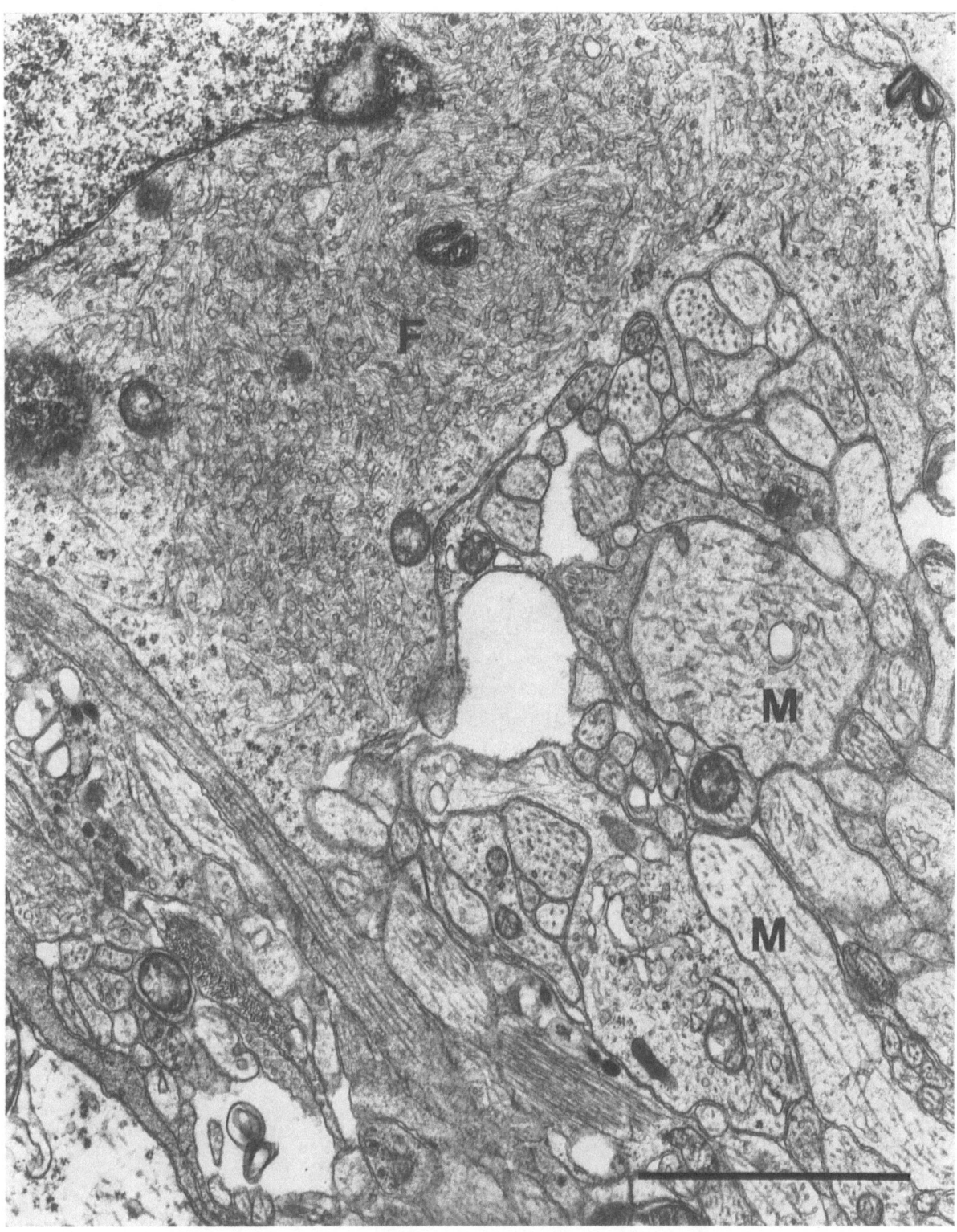

Fig. 10.4. *Medulloblastoma.* Even when the tumour is predominantly primitive in appearance, occasional medullo-blastoma cells containing randomly orientated 6- to 9-nm glial filaments (*F*) may be found, as in the *upper part* of this field. Such glial differentiation may rarely be very marked, with numerous swollen tumour cells entirely filled by glial filaments. The processes of more typical medulloblastoma cells contain 20-nm microtubules (*M*), as seen on the *right*. (Bar = 2 μm)

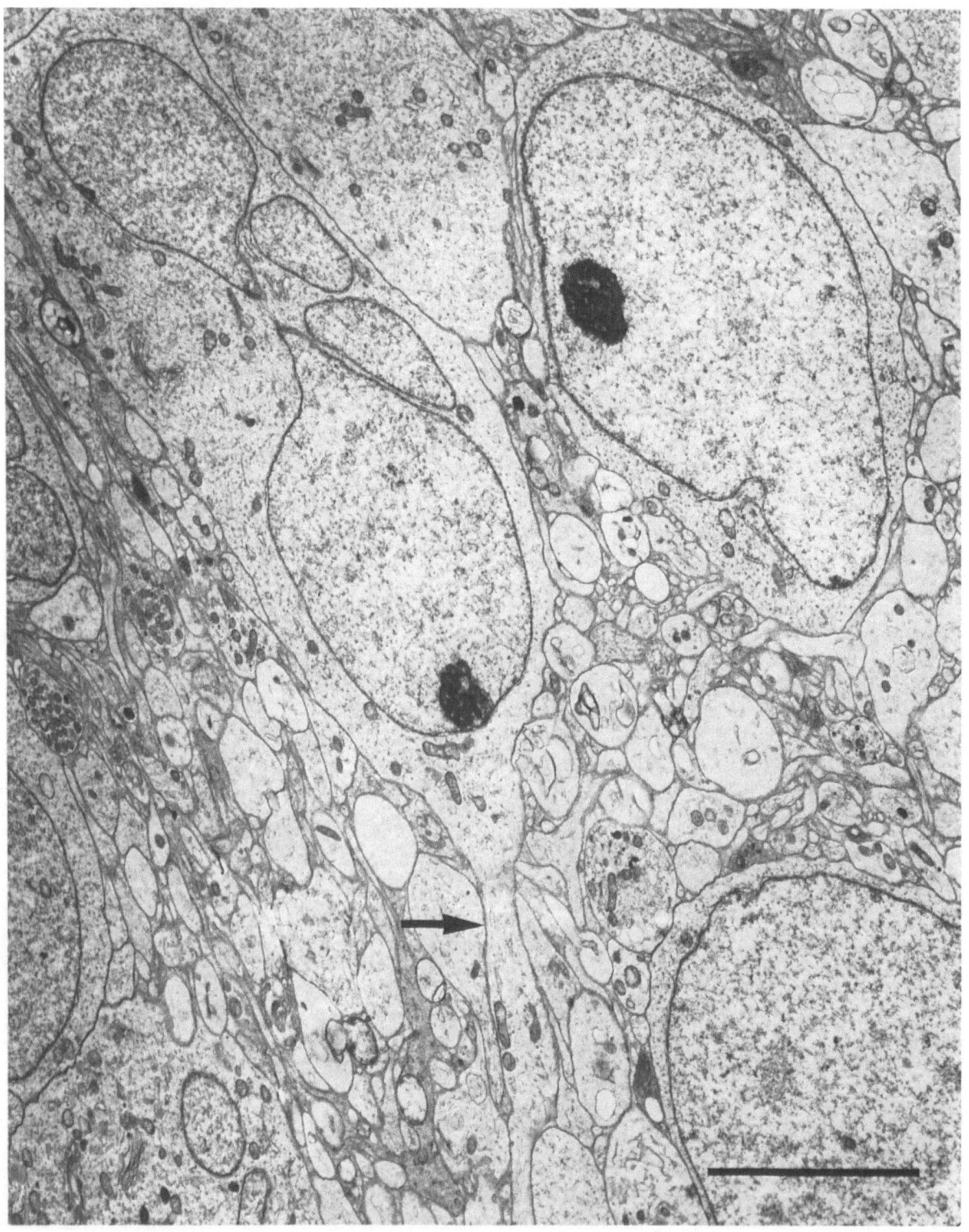

Fig. 10.5. *Medulloblastoma.* Many largely primitive medulloblastomas also contain scattered unipolar cells, like that in the *centre*. These cells have prominent nucleoli and tapering terminal cell processes (*arrow*), suggesting neuroblastic differentiation. Evidence of glial differentiation may be present in the same tumour, indicating a bipotential differentiating capacity. (Bar = 5 μm)

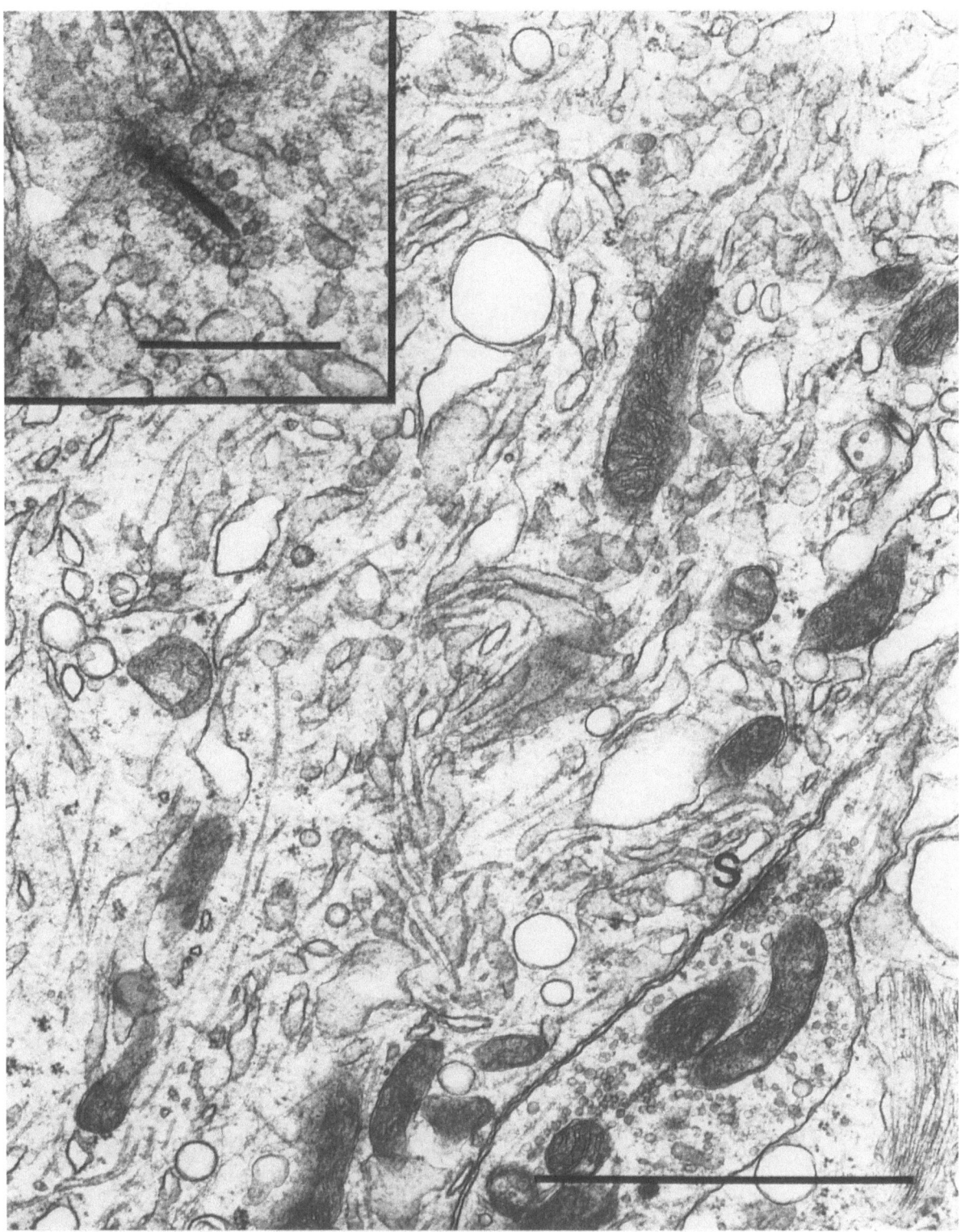

Fig. 10.6. *Medulloblastoma.* Very rarely, medulloblastomas may show frank ganglionic differentiation, as here, with swollen cell bodies filled by 20-nm microtubules and forming synapses (*S*) with adjacent processes. (Bar = 2 µm) *Inset*: Other specialised neuroblastic organelles may also be found in these cases, such as this synaptic ("vesicle-crowned") lamella, normally a feature of retinoblastomas. (Bar = 0.5 µm)

11 Central Neuroblastoma

Neuroblastomas were not initially thought to occur as primary central nervous system tumours, and although now well documented, they still remain rare and rather controversial neoplasms in this site. The ultrastructural features are very similar to those of peripheral neuroblastomas, the main difference being the absence of connective tissue elements between cells. Central neuroblastomas also show ultrastructural similarities with other neuroblastic tumours of the central nervous system, such as primary pineal tumours and medulloblastomas with ganglionic differentiation.

The tumour cell bodies have a polygonal or spherical shape and are usually closely packed together in clumps. The nuclei are large and rounded, with finely granular chromatin and occasional prominent nucleoli. There is typically only a scanty rim of perinuclear cytoplasm, which contains abundant polyribosomes but sparse endoplasmic reticulum and other organelles. Numerous, thin, electron-lucent cell processes are also present, and form an interlacing meshwork between groups of cell bodies. They often resemble immature neuritic processes, and contain longitudinally orientated 10-nm neurofilaments and 20-nm microtubules. Desmosome-type junctions may be present between cell bodies, but are more often found between their peripheral processes. The extracellular space is usually scanty, and contains amorphous ground substance but no collagen or other connective tissue elements.

In addition to these general features, most cases also show definite evidence of neuronal differentiation in some of the tumour cell bodies and processes, confirming the neuroblastic nature of the tumour. Dense-core vesicles are often present, and are more often found in cell processes than in perinuclear cytoplasm. Their outer diameter varies from 70 to 170 nm and some examples may appear empty, lacking the central dense granule. Smaller 35- to 40-nm diameter synaptic vesicles also occur chiefly in the cell processes, and may form synaptic complexes alongside desmosome-like membrane thickenings. Although not widely described in these tumours, non-motile, neuronal-type cilia may also be found, usually buried within tumour cell bodies. Neuroblastic rosettes, when present, are formed ultrastructurally from an outer rim of cell bodies with numerous, thin, centrally directed processes which contain dense-core vesicles. Scattered cells and processes containing bundles of 6- to 9-nm glial filaments are also often present in these tumours, in contrast to peripheral neuroblastomas. It is uncertain whether these fibrillar elements represent divergent glial differentiation in neuroblastoma cells, or are simply pre-existing, reactive astrocytes trapped within the tumour.

Further Reading

Azzarelli B, Richards O, Anton AH, Roessmann U (1977) Central neuroblastoma. Electron microscopic observations and catecholamine determinations. J Neuropathol Exp Neurol 36: 384–397

Grisoli F, Vincentelli F, Boudouresques G, Delpuech F, Hassoun J, Raybaud C (1981) Primary cerebral neuroblastoma in an adult man. Surg Neurol 16: 266–270

Rhodes RH, David RL, Kassel SH, Clague BH (1978) Primary cerebral neuroblastoma: a light and electron microscopic study. Acta Neuropathol 41: 119–124

Shin WY, Laufer H, Lee YC, Aftalion B, Hirano A, Zimmermann HM (1978) Fine structure of a cerebellar neuroblastoma. Acta Neuropathol 42: 11–13

Yagishita S, Itoh Y, Chiba Y, Yamishita T, Nakazima F, Kuwabara T (1980) Cerebellar neuroblastoma. A light and ultrastructural study. Acta Neuropathol 50: 139–142

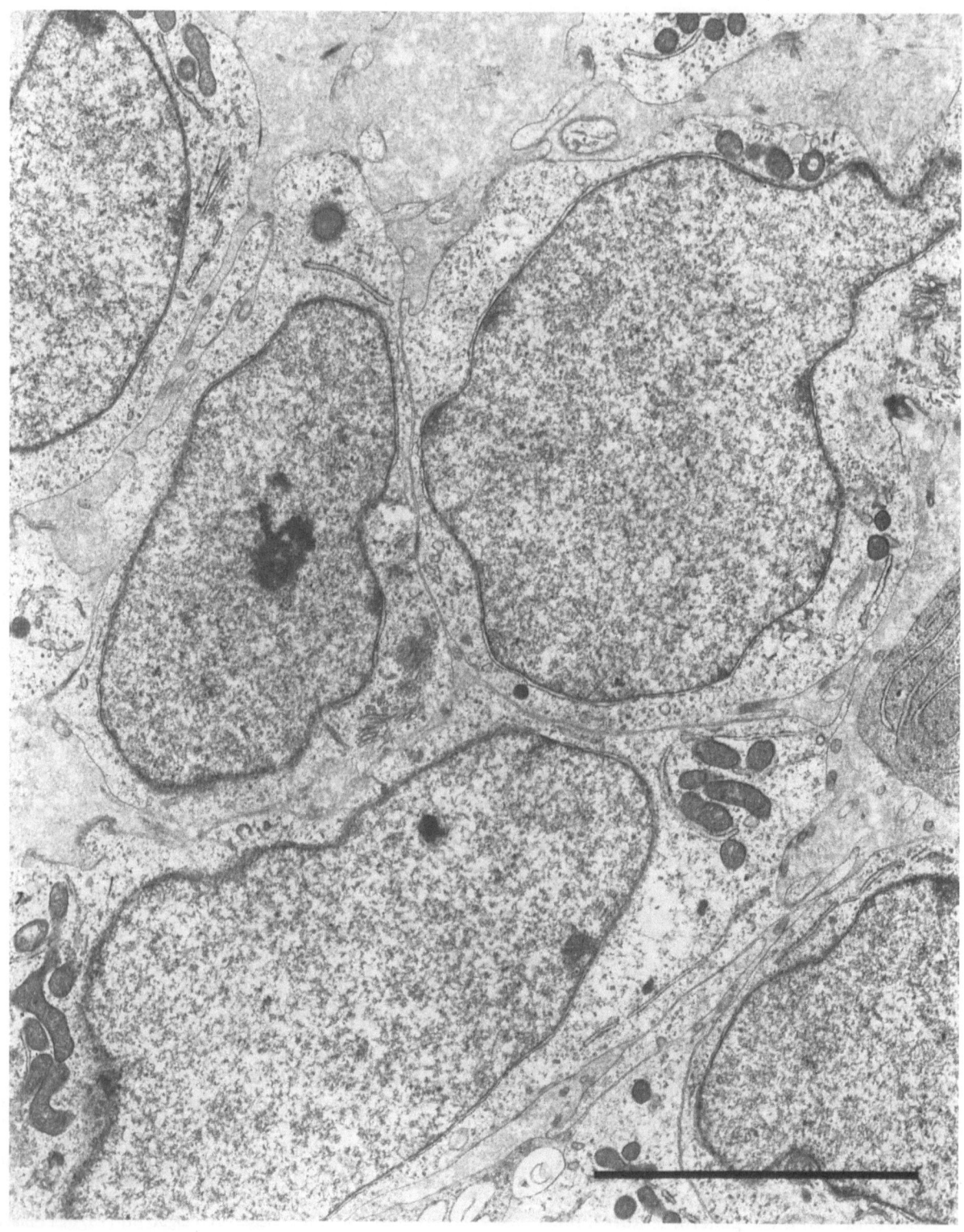

Fig. 11.1. *Central neuroblastoma.* The cells tend to be closely packed together in small groups, as in this field, and have irregularly rounded nuclei with finely granular chromatin and occasional nucleoli. There is normally only a scanty rim of perinuclear cytoplasm, which contains chiefly polyribosomes. The extracellular space is filled by amorphous matrix, like that seen at the *top*, and does not contain collagen or other connective tissue elements. (Bar = 5 μm)

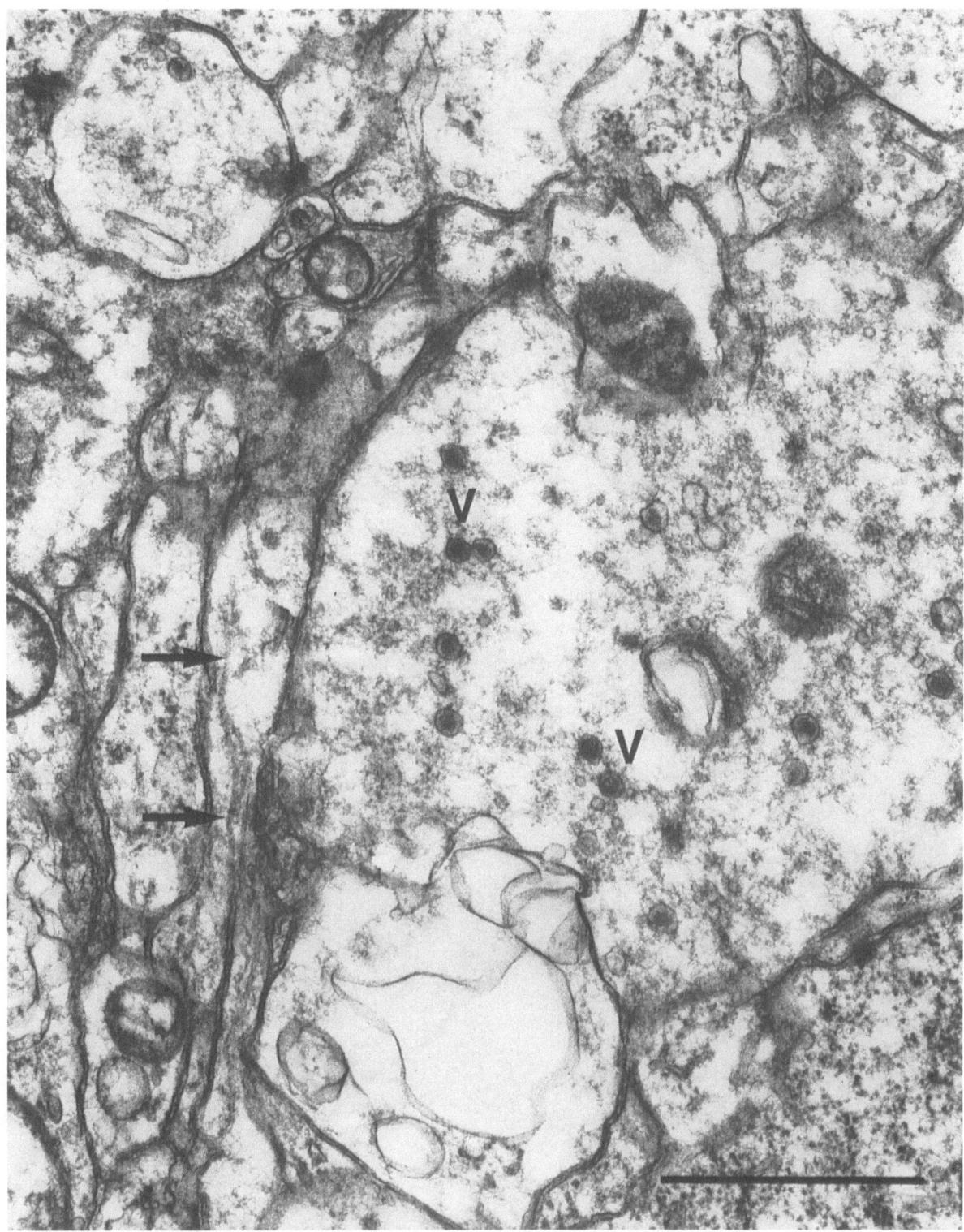

Fig. 11.2. *Central neuroblastoma.* The thin, electron-lucent cell processes resemble neuritic processes and form an intricate meshwork. They usually contain longitudinally orientated 20-nm microtubules (*arrows*). Dense-core vesicles (*V*) may also be present and have an outer diameter varying between 70 and 170 nm. Some examples may appear empty and lack a central dense granule. (Bar = 1 μm)

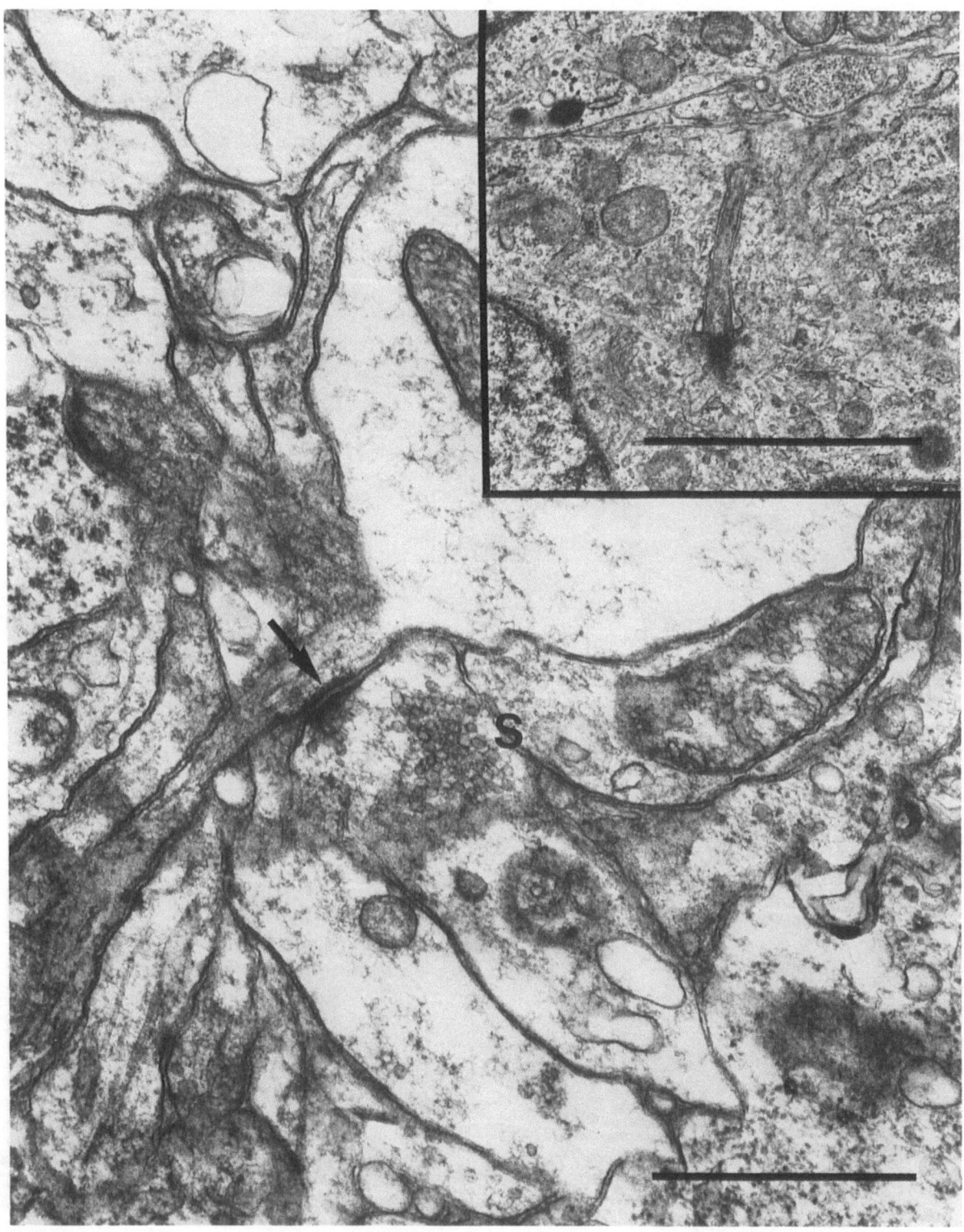

Fig. 11.3. *Central neuroblastoma.* In well-differentiated examples, the tumour cell processes contain 35- to 40-nm diameter synaptic vesicles (*S*). These may aggregate around desmosome-like membrane thickenings to form synaptic complexes (*arrow*). (Bar = 1 μm) *Inset*: Non-motile, neuronal-type cilia are rare and tend to be buried within tumour cell bodies, as in this case. (Bar = 2 μm)

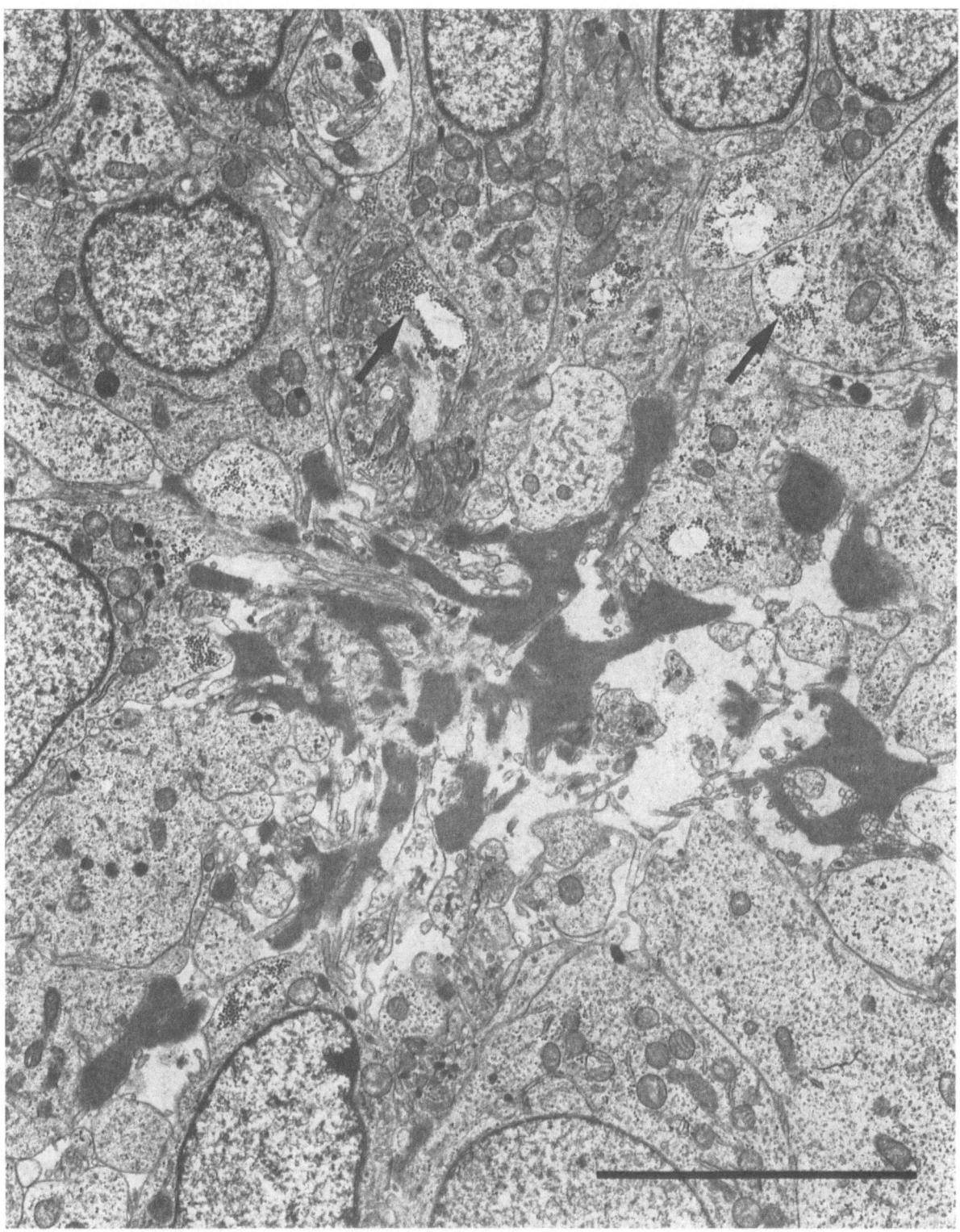

Fig. 11.4. *Central neuroblastoma.* Neuroblastic rosettes are formed from an outer circle of tumour cell bodies with numerous, thin, centrally directed processes containing dense-core vesicles. The central area of one such rosette is illustrated here. In this tumour the cells were unusual in containing pools of glycogen granules within their perikaryal cytoplasm (*arrows*). (Bar = 5 μm)

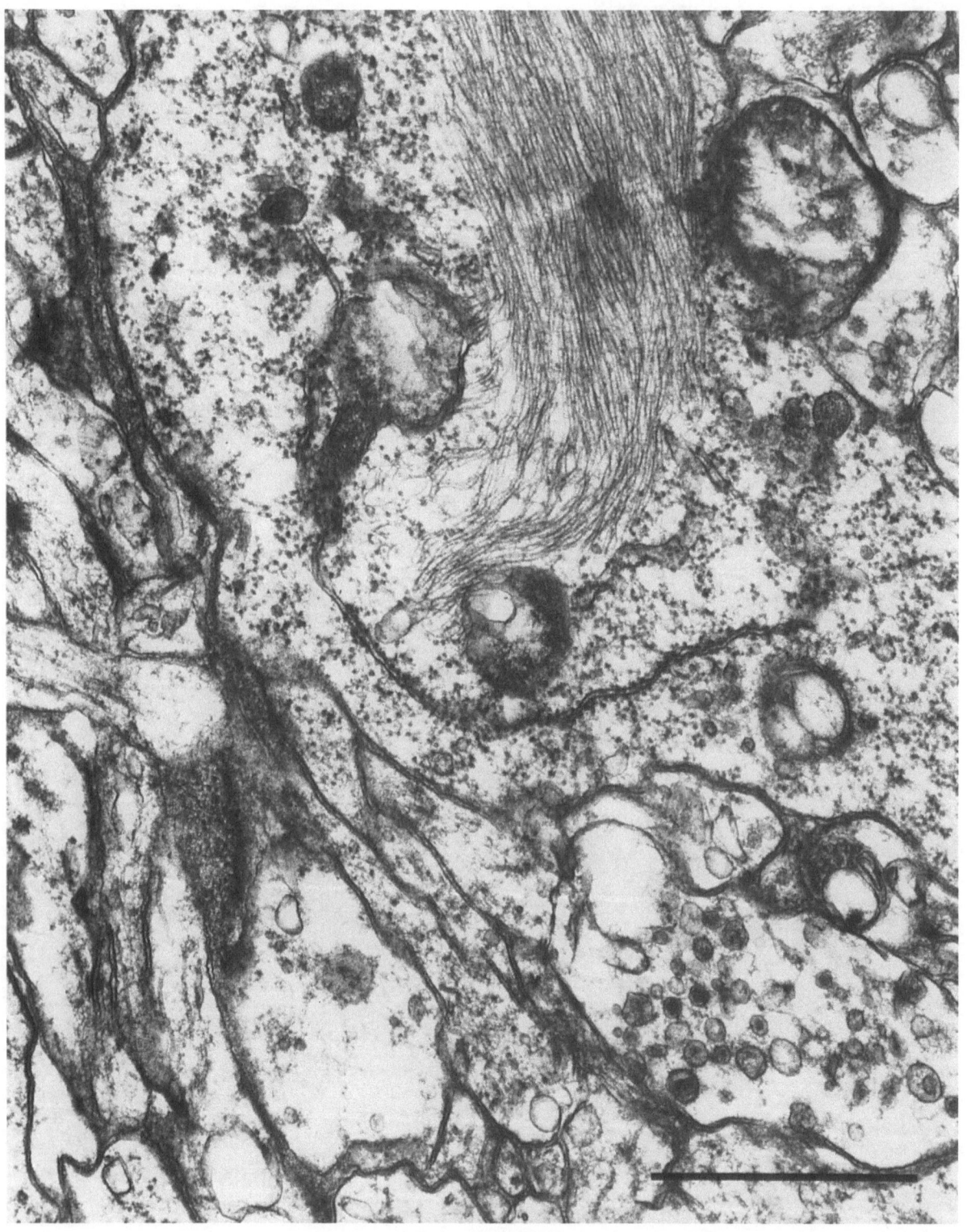

Fig. 11.5. *Central neuroblastoma.* Cells and processes containing 6- to 9-nm glial filaments are often scattered through these tumours, and one such process can be seen at the *top* of this figure. It is not certain whether these represent divergent astrocytic differentiation, or are simply pre-existing reactive glial elements trapped within the tumour. (Bar = 1 μm)

12 Ganglioglioma

Gangliogliomas are rare tumours that are ultrastructurally similar to central ganglioneuromas but have an unequivocally neoplastic glial component in addition to the ganglionic elements. Typical examples consist of a complex loose meshwork of large, often bizarre tumour cell bodies and irregular processes, sometimes interspersed with degenerating elements of the infiltrated neuropil. One tumour cell type resembles a neoplastic ganglion cell, and often has a unipolar arrangement with a single terminal process. The nuclei of these cells have a rounded outline, finely granular chromatin and prominent nucleoli. The perikaryal cytoplasm is voluminous and contains abundant organelles, including 10-nm neurofilaments, lipofuscin granules and prominent cisternae of rough endoplasmic reticulum. In addition, there may be numerous dense-core vesicles, usually less than 220 nm in diameter, and also larger membrane-bound structures up to 400 nm across. These larger structures resemble dense-core vesicles but have a concentric, lamellar core. Similar bodies have been described in the stumps of experimentally severed axons, and they are thought to represent degenerating dense-core vesicles. Cell processes associated with the neoplastic ganglion cells often resemble unmyelinated axons and contain 10-nm neurofilaments, 20-nm microtubules and dense-core vesicles. Smaller, 35- to 40-nm synaptic vesicles and well-formed synaptic complexes may also be present.

The other main cell type resembles a swollen neoplastic astrocyte. The nucleus is typically highly convoluted with clumped chromatin, and is often flattened against one side of the cell body. Perikaryal cytoplasm is again abundant and is largely packed with dense bundles of 6- to 9-nm glial filaments, although there may be other, scattered organelles, including occasional dense-core vesicles. Rosenthal bodies are sometimes seen in association with the filaments (see Chap. 1). The numerous irregular processes of these cells are also packed with filaments and do not form synapses like the ganglionic processes.

Some reports have also described a third, mesenchymal cell type with a basement membrane, which is closely associated with collagen fibrils and resembles a ganglionic satellite cell. On the basis of these cells and the ganglionic morphology of the neoplastic neuronal cells, it has been suggested that these tumours show ultrastructural similarities with sympathetic ganglia and may originate from autonomic nervous system hamartomas occurring within the central nervous system.

Further Reading

Lee JC, Glasauer FE (1968) Ganglioglioma: light and electron microscopic study. Neurochir (Stuttg) 11: 160–170

Robertson DM, Hendry WS, Vogel FS (1964) Central ganglioneuroma: a case study using electron microscopy. J Neuropathol Exp Neurol 23: 692–705

Rubinstein LJ, Herman MM (1972) A light and electron microscopic study of a temporal lobe ganglioglioma. J Neurol Sci 16: 27–28

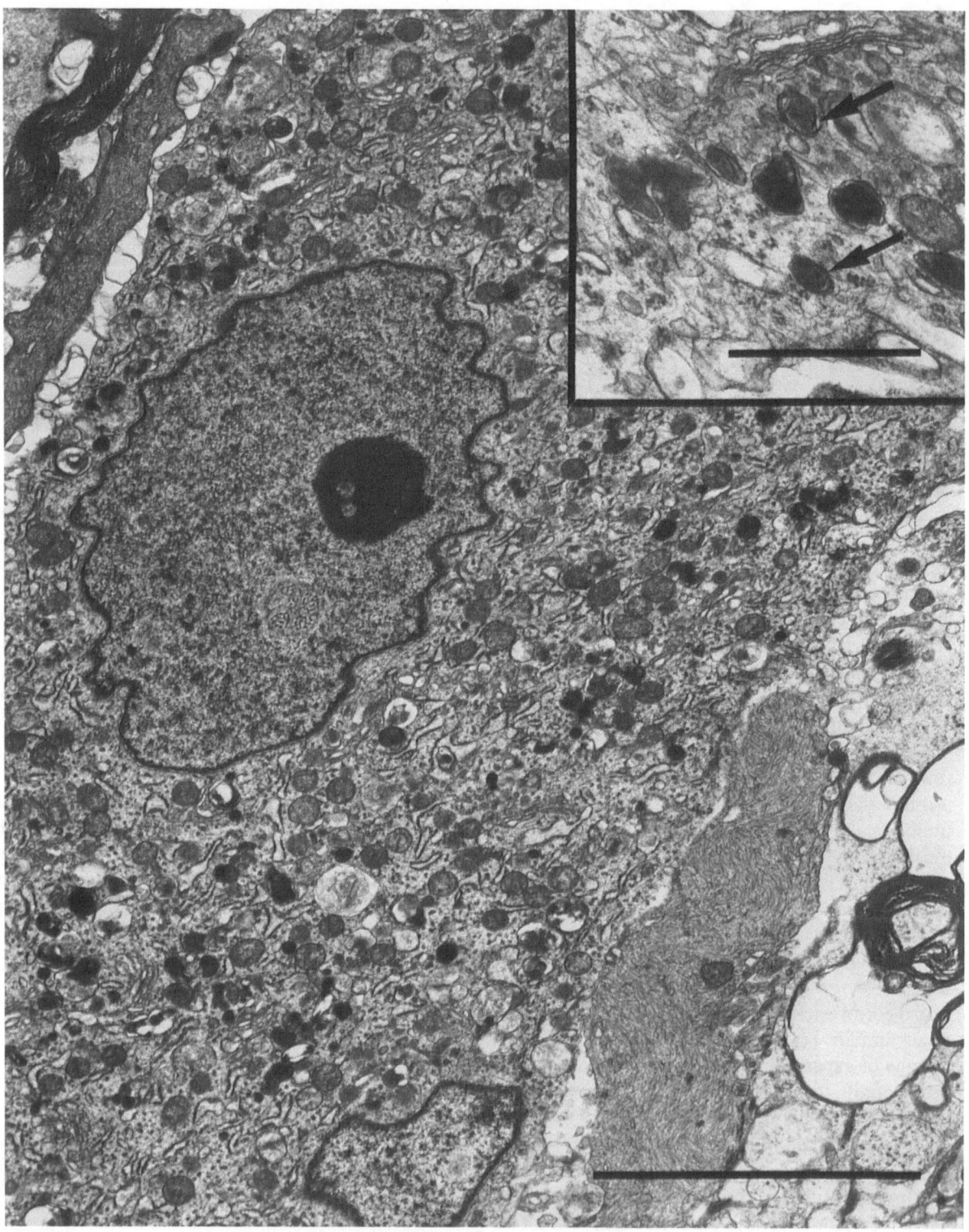

Fig. 12.1. *Ganglioglioma.* One type of cell present in these tumours resembles a neoplastic ganglion cell, like the example shown here. The nuclei of these cells have finely granular chromatin and prominent nucleoli. Their voluminous cytoplasm usually contains abundant organelles, including cisternae of rough endoplasmic reticulum and typical dense-core vesicles. (Bar = 5 μm) *Inset*: Some of these cells also contain larger membrane-bound organelles up to 400 nm across. These structures often have a concentric, lamellar core (*arrows*), and probably represent degenerating dense-core vesicles. (Bar = 1 μm)

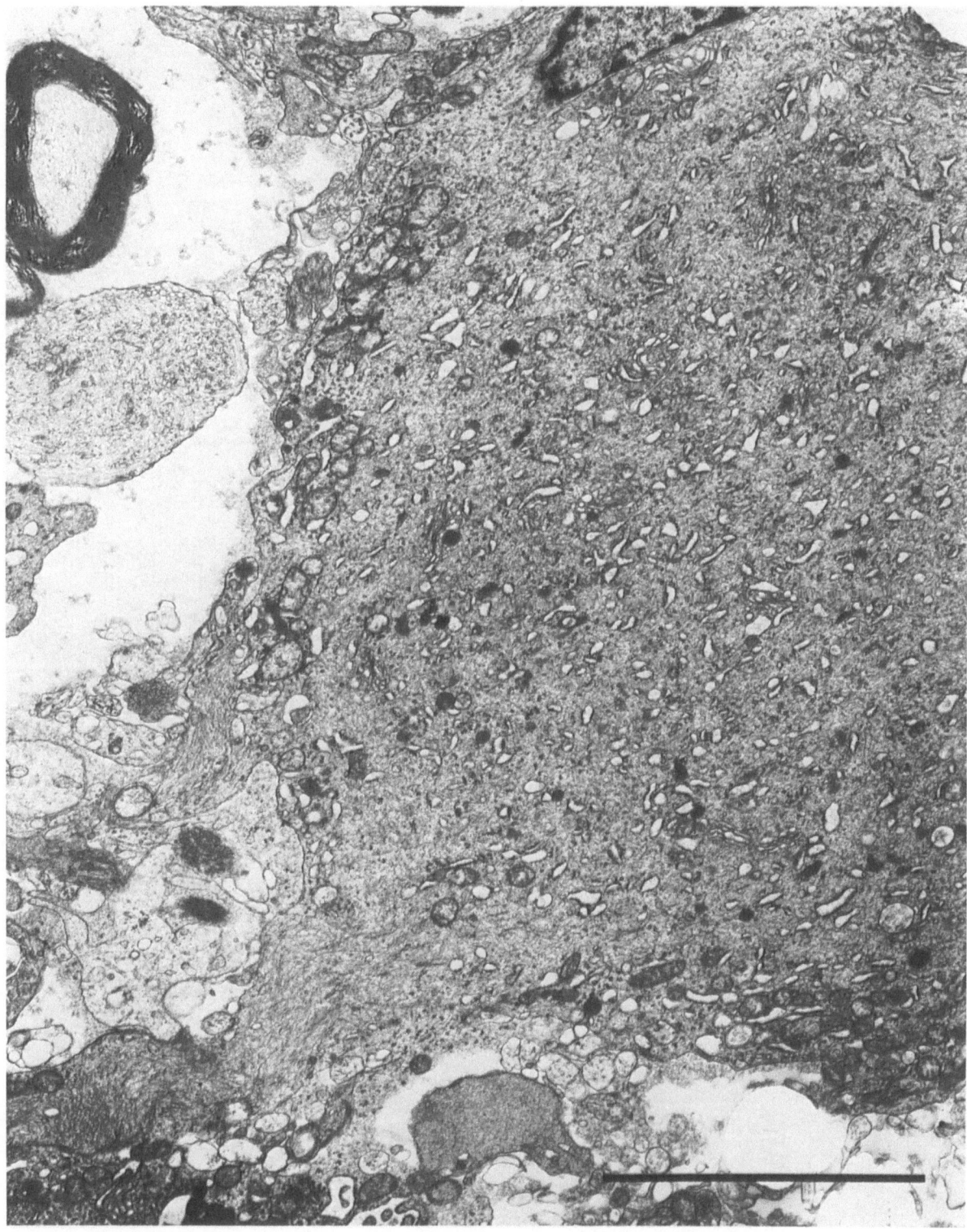

Fig. 12.2. *Ganglioglioma.* The other main cell type is illustrated here and resembles a bizarre neoplastic astrocyte. The nuclei of these cells have clumped chromatin, and are often flattened against the periphery of the cell body. The cell bodies contain scattered organelles, including dense-core vesicles, but both the voluminous cytoplasm and peripheral processes are largely filled by 6- to 9-nm glial filaments, as in this case. (Bar = 5 μm)

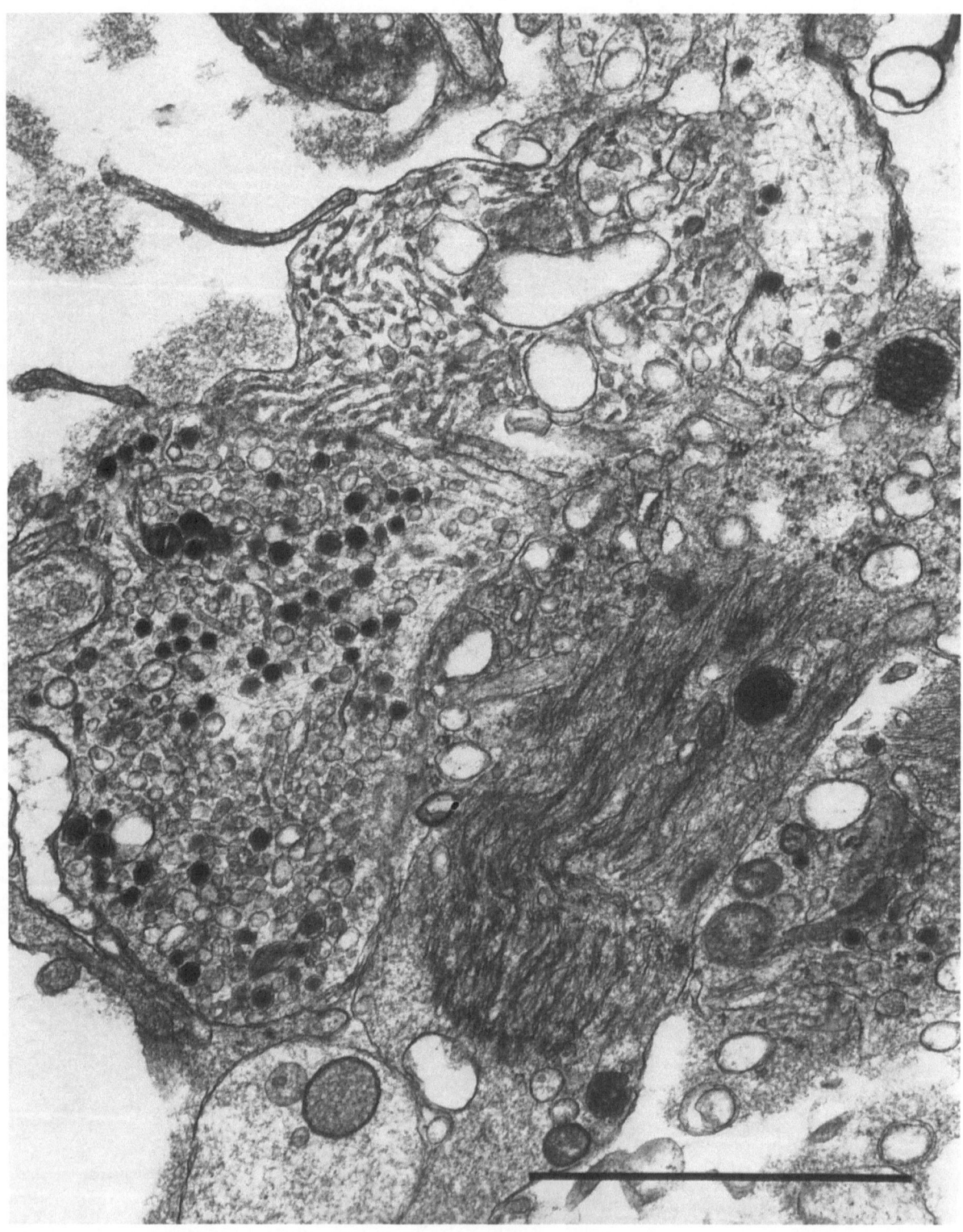

Fig. 12.3. *Ganglioglioma.* Ganglionic cell processes, like that on the *left*, contain dense-core vesicles up to 220 nm across and smaller, 35- to 40-nm diameter synaptic vesicles. In some instances well-formed synapses may also be present. Neoplastic astrocyte processes, like the one on the *right*, are largely filled by 6- to 9-nm glial filaments. (Bar = 2 μm)

13 Meningioma

The main features of all non-vasoformative meningiomas are similar at electron microscopic level, although there is variation in the relative predominance of fibroblastic and syncytial components. The tumour cells have many ultrastructural features in common with non-neoplastic arachnoidal cells, from which they are presumed to take origin. Their cytoplasm is electron lucent, and contains generally sparse organelles but abundant 10-nm filaments, which extend into tenuous processes. The cells lack basement membrane.

In fibroblastic areas, tumour cells are mainly spindle shaped with flattened nuclei. They typically form parallel arrays, with closely dovetailed palisades of elongate cell processes. The extracellular space may contain abundant collagen, but there is no evidence that this is produced by the tumour cells themselves. Some reports have described interspersed, darker-staining cells with abundant rough endoplasmic reticulum, and these may represent the fibroblasts responsible for the collagen production.

In more syncytial areas, tumour cells have plump cell bodies and rounded nuclei, which may show deep invaginations. The cell bodies are tightly juxtaposed and linked by numerous, prominent desmosomes. There is little free extracellular space, and collagen is not usually present. The cells typically contain abundant mitochondria, and the 10-nm filaments in their cytoplasm may have a whorled pattern. The long, thin cell processes often show a characteristic "jigsaw" type of interlocking pattern, but may also be arranged in concentric bundles around central cell bodies to form whorls.

Psammoma bodies have a central core consisting of collagen interspersed with amorphous or filamentous material, and are again surrounded by concentric lamellae of cell processes. In more mature examples, the core contains increasing amounts of osmiophilic, calcified material, and the surrounding processes may have a degenerate, vacuolated appearance. The plasma membrane of the innermost process is often incomplete, and intracellular elements, especially 10-nm filaments, appear continuous with those in the central core. Psammoma bodies are thought to be derived from a combination of amorphous, proteinaceous material secreted by the surrounding cells and the degenerated elements of central tumour cell bodies. In some instances a similar arrangement of degenerating processes may be found around an intact central capillary blood vessel, rather than a psammomatous core.

In microcystic meningiomas, the tumour cells have a stellate appearance and are widely separated by large loculi of extracellular space containing scanty collagen. These extracellular loculi, or microcysts, are enclosed by tenuous cell processes, often linked by desmosomes.

Further Reading

Cervós-Navarro J, Vasquez JJ (1969) An electron microscopic study of meningiomas. Acta Neuropathol 13: 301–323

Gonatus NK, Besen M (1963) An electron microscopic study of three human psammomatous meningiomas. J Neuropathol Exp Neurol 22: 263–273

Kepes J (1961) Electron microscopic studies of meningiomas. Am J Pathol 39: 499–510

Napolitano L, Kyle R, Fisher ER (1963) Ultrastructure of meningiomas and the derivation and nature of their cellular components. Cancer 17: 233–241

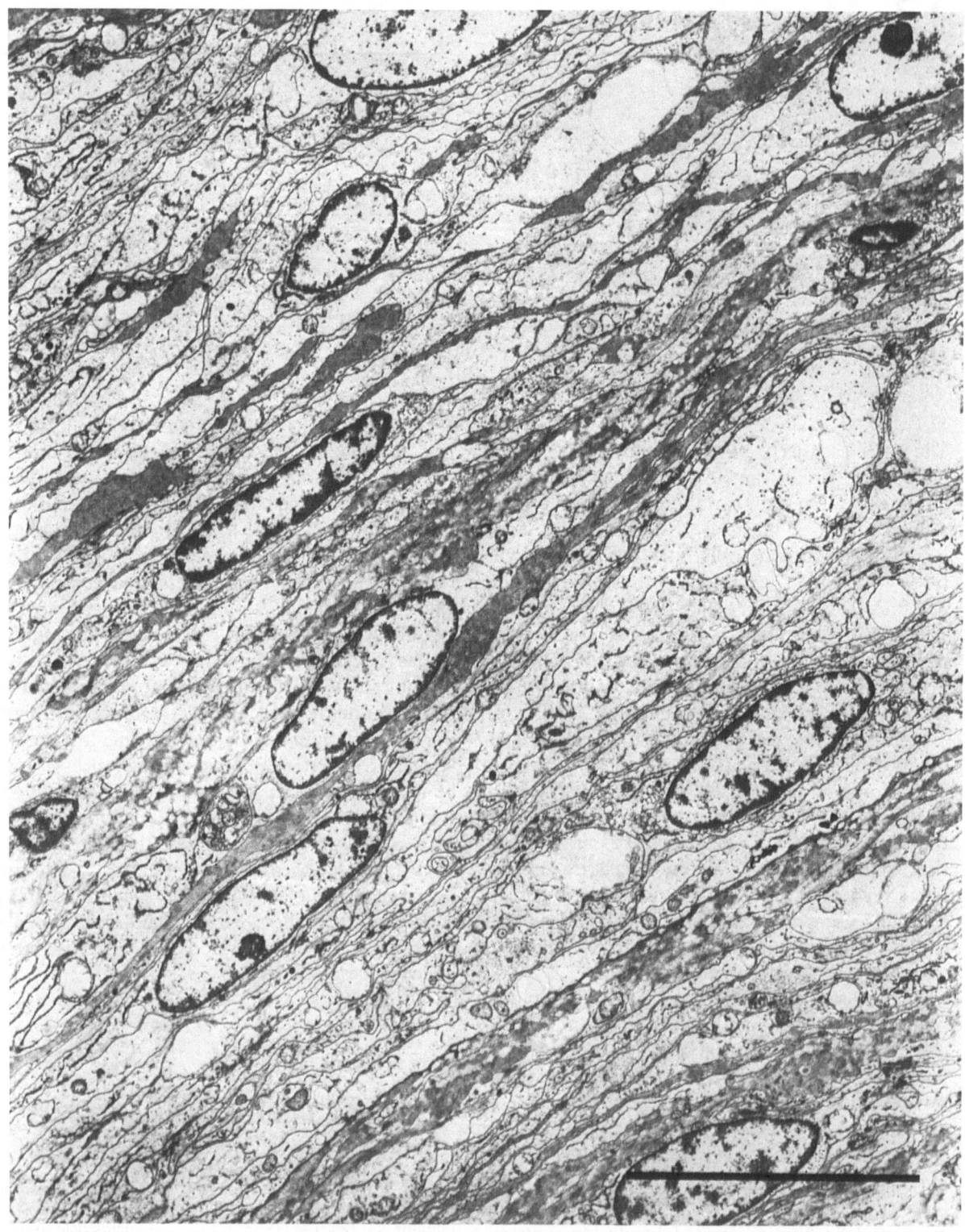

Fig. 13.1. *Meningioma.* In fibroblastic areas, like that shown here, the cells are mostly spindle shaped with flattened nuclei. They form parallel arrays, with palisades of closely dovetailed, elongate processes. At higher magnifications the darker-staining extracellular spaces can be seen to contain abundant collagen. (Bar = 10 μm)

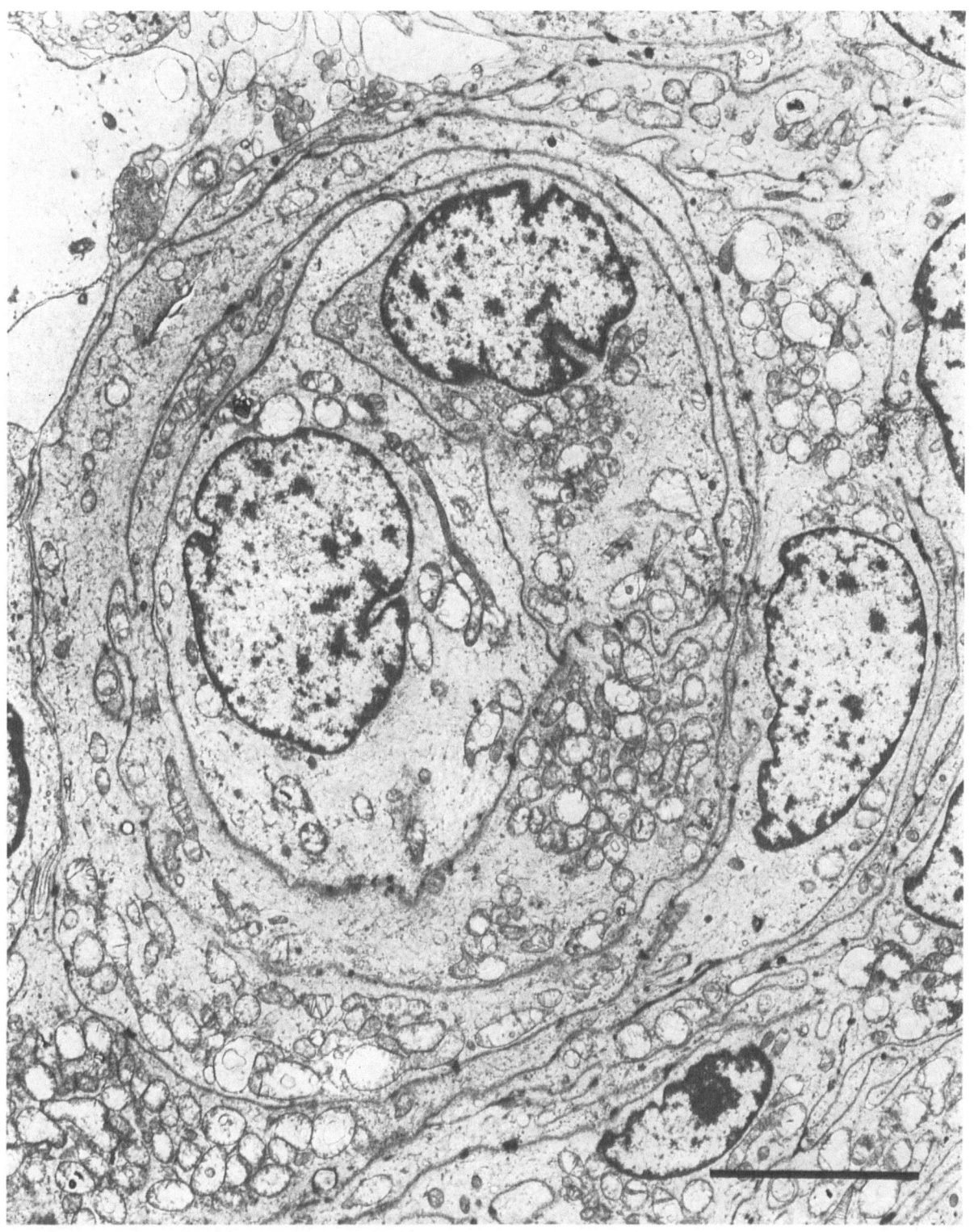

Fig. 13.2. *Meningioma.* In syncytial areas, the tumour cells are mostly plump with rounded or superficially invaginated nuclei, as in this figure. The cells are closely linked by numerous desmosomes, visible only as black dots at this magnification, and may contain abundant mitochondria. Whorls, like the one illustrated here, are usually formed from central cell bodies surrounded by concentric bundles of cell processes. (Bar = 5 μm)

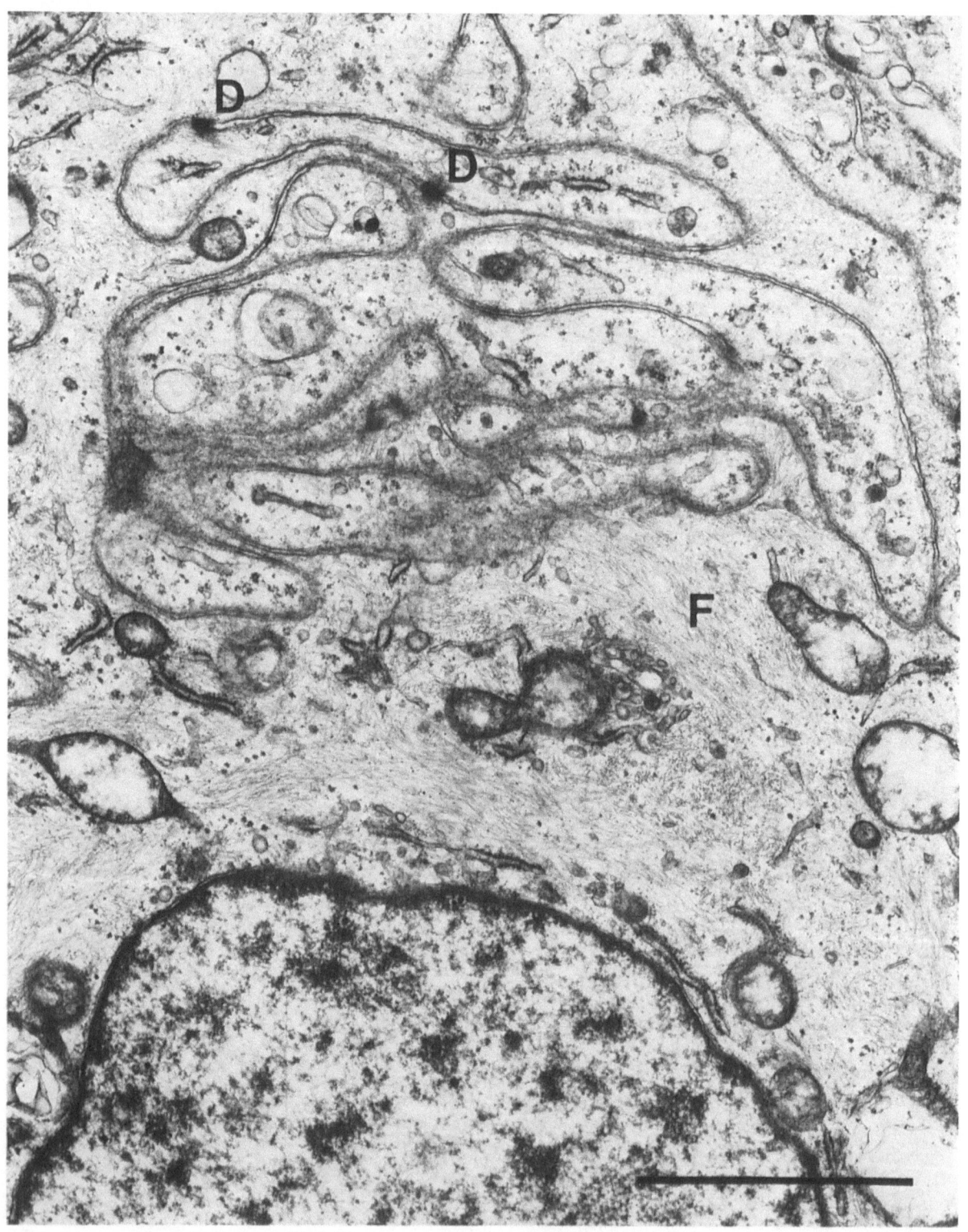

Fig. 13.3. *Meningioma.* Tumour cell bodies and processes have electron-lucent cytoplasm and contain abundant 10-nm filaments (*F*). In syncytial areas, the cell processes often form a characteristic "jigsaw" or interlocking pattern, as seen at the *top* of this figure, and are linked by desmosomes (*D*). (Bar = 2 μm)

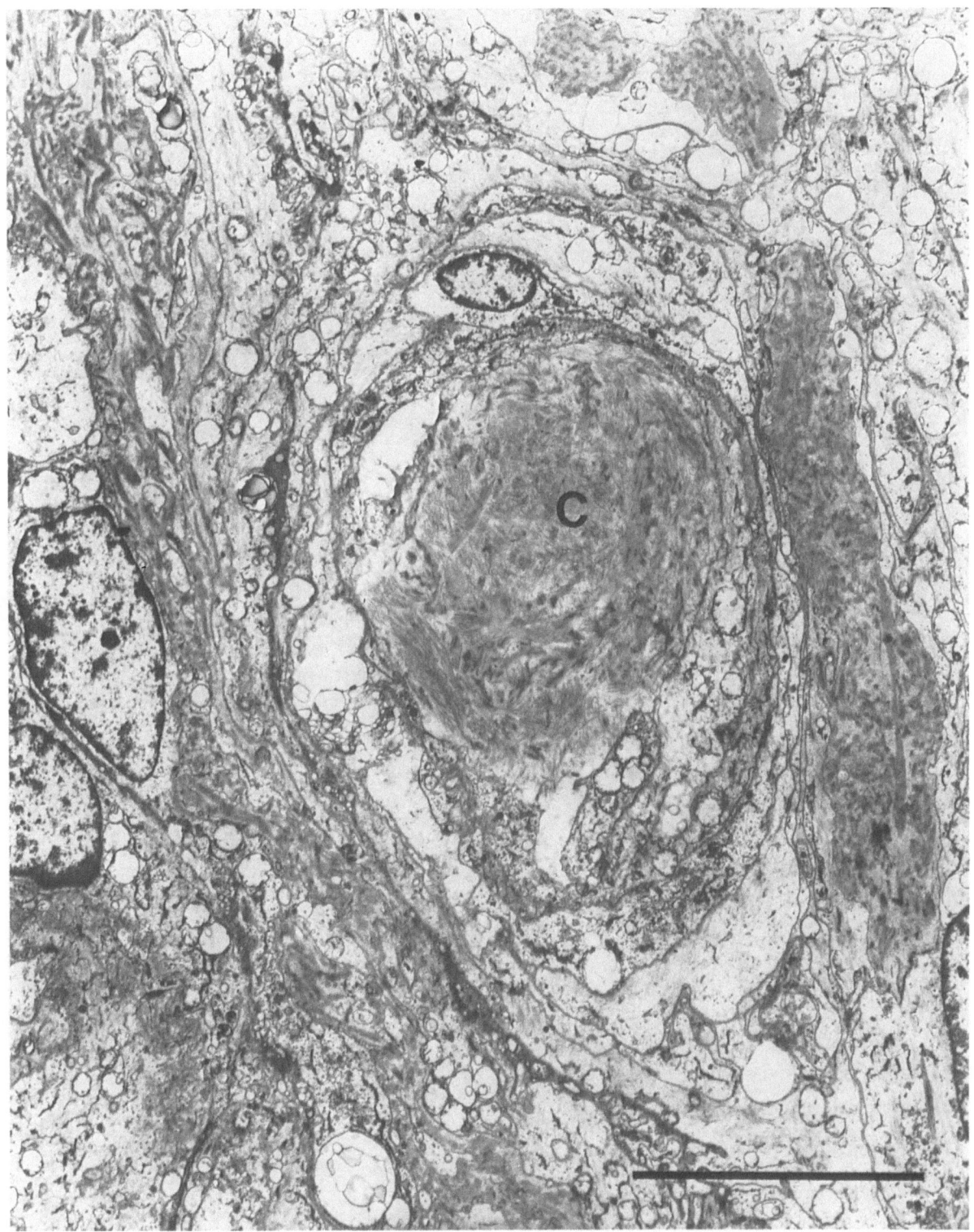

Fig. 13.4. *Meningioma.* Psammoma bodies have a central core (*C*) consisting of collagen mixed with filamentous and granular material. This is surrounded by concentric lamellae of degenerate-looking, vacuolated cell processes. Better developed examples than the one shown here also contain increasing amounts of osmiophilic, calcified material. (Bar = 10 μm)

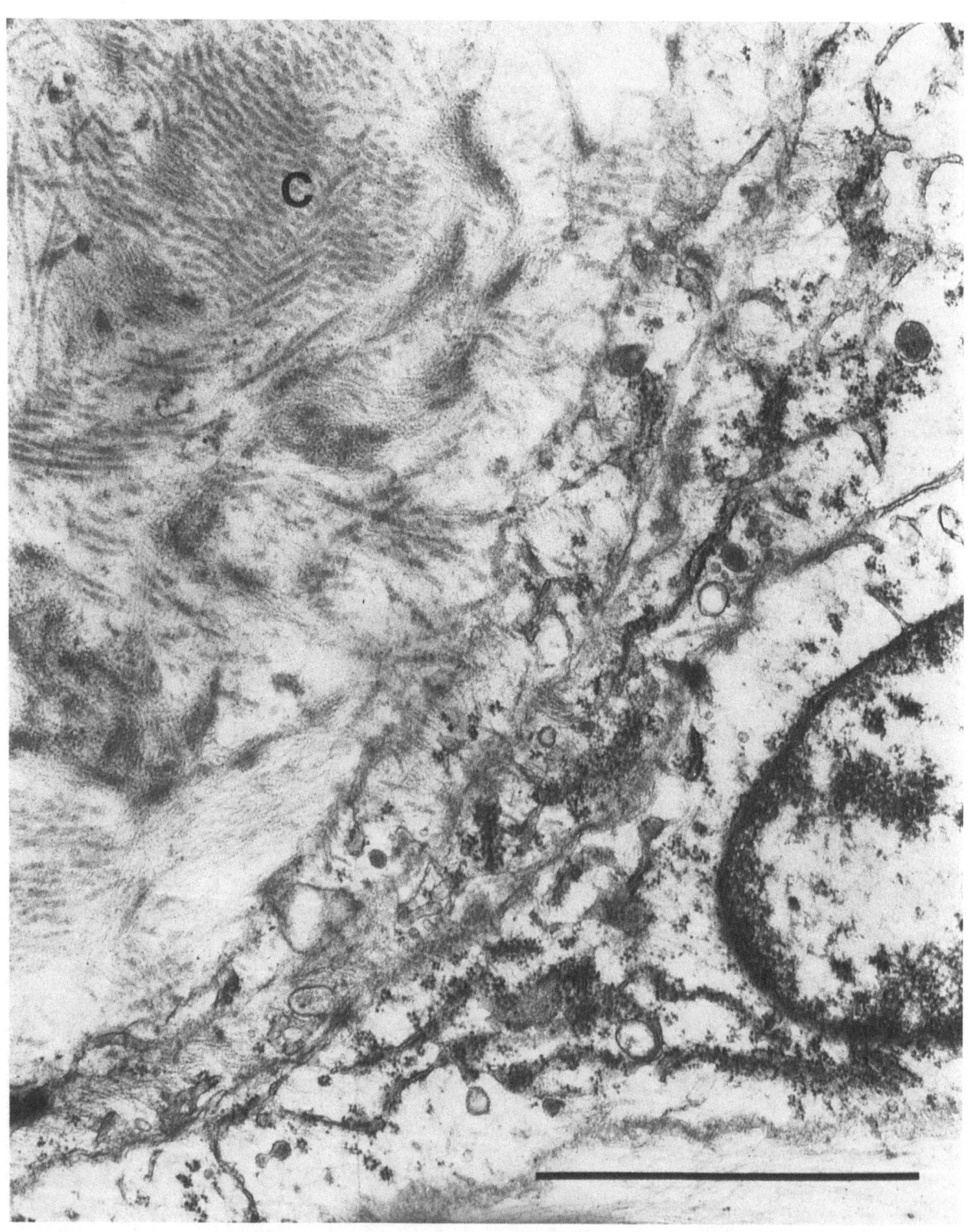

Fig. 13.5. *Meningioma.* The plasma membrane of the innermost concentric cell process around psammoma bodies is often incomplete or entirely absent, as can be seen in the *centre* of this figure. The intracellular filaments of such degenerate processes often appear to merge with the filaments in the central core of the psammoma body, which occupies the *top left* of the field shown here. The core is thought to be formed from degenerated elements of central cell bodies together with proteinaceous amorphous cell secretions, but abundant collagen is also present (*C*). (Bar = 2 μm)

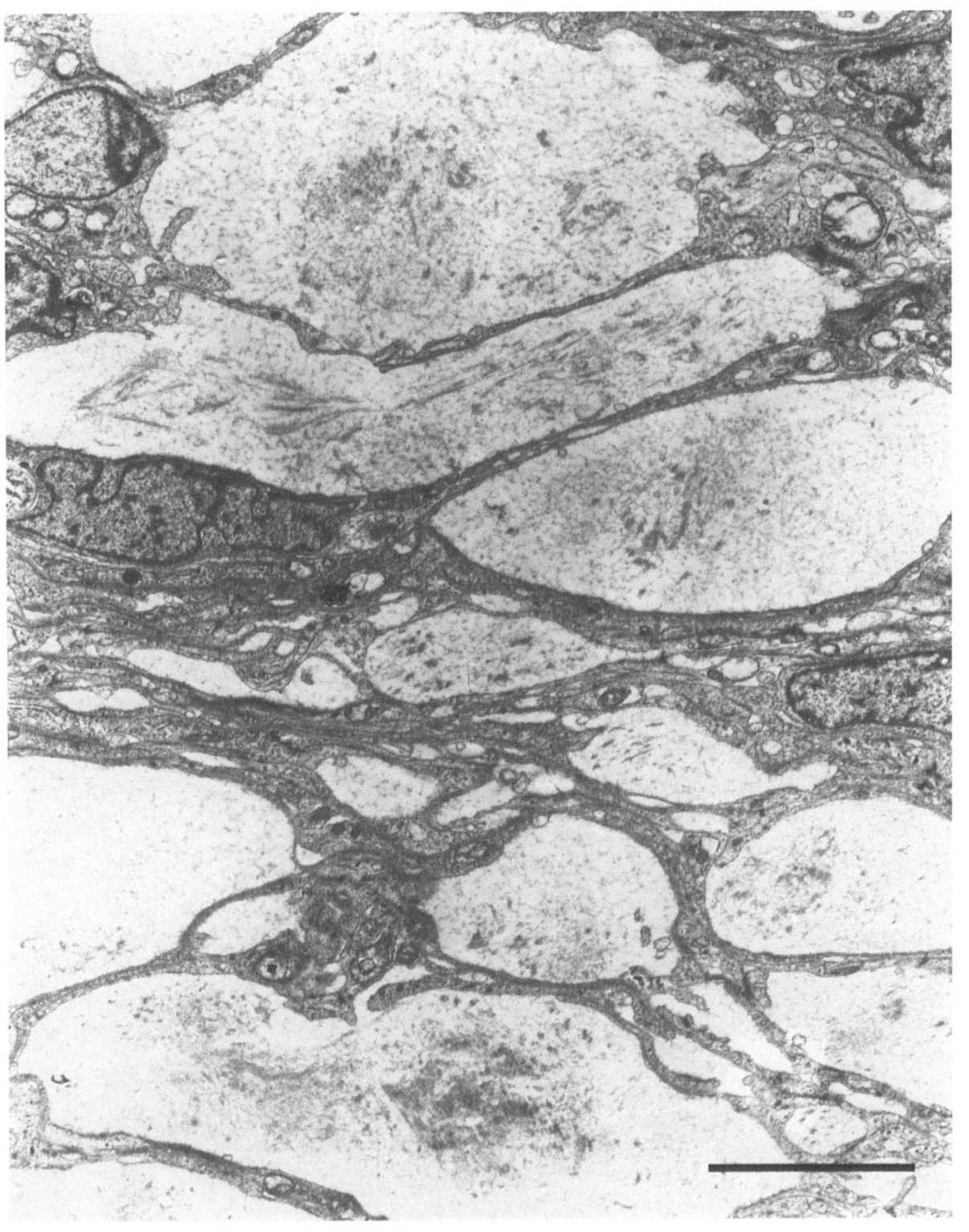

Fig. 13.6. *Microcystic meningioma.* In this tumour variant the cells have a stellate appearance and are separated by large loculi of extracellular space, like those illustrated here. These loculi, or "microcysts", are enclosed by tenuous cell processes and contain scanty collagen. (Bar = 5 μm)

14 Vasoformative Meningioma

The ultrastructural features of this group of tumours suggest that they are distinct from other meningiomas and possibly derived from blood vessel elements, such as pericytes, rather than arachnoidal cells. The various different subgroups proposed for vasoformative meningiomas are not clearly defined at ultrastructural level, and there appears to be a spectrum between the relatively well differentiated, or angioblastic types and the more malignant, haemangiopericytic forms.

The angioblastic types of tumour show some ultrastructural similarities with haemangioblastomas, and are formed from sheets of uniform, plump, polygonal cells with central, rounded nuclei and prominent nucleoli. Like the cells of both haemangioblastomas and syncytial meningiomas, there is abundant electron lucent cytoplasm, largely filled with bundles of 10-nm filaments, and no distinct basement membranes are present round the cell bodies. Unlike syncytial meningiomas, however, the cells show little tendency to form peripheral processes, and desmosomes are scarce or entirely absent. There is no collagen between the cells, and the extracellular space is filled with electron-dense, amorphous matrix. The matrix is especially prominent in the wide perivascular spaces, where it resembles abnormal basement membrane material. The abundant capillaries are usually thin walled, with fenestrated endothelial cells which appear morphologically distinct from the tumour cells.

Towards the haemangiopericytic end of the spectrum, the tumours show an increasing ultrastructural resemblance to haemangiopericytomas elsewhere in the body, thus supporting the concept of an origin from pericytes. Pleomorphic tumour cells with large, irregular nuclei are tightly packed together in clumps, often deeply indenting each other. The cells form irregular, short processes, and there may also be tightly interlocking microvillous processes between cell bodies. The cytoplasm is usually electron lucent and contains mixed organelles, including abundant polyribosomes and bundles of 10-nm filaments. Periodic densities have been found in filamentous areas, raising the possibility of smooth muscle differentiation. There is little extracellular space between adjacent cells, but desmosome junctions are not usually found. The numerous abnormal vascular channels are formed from irregular, plump cells similar to the tumour cells, and lack fenestrations or a typical endothelial lining. The vessel lumina are often very narrow and sometimes appear to be entirely obliterated, leaving discrete, rounded clumps of cells. These are separated from the surrounding tumour tissue only by a narrow zone of electron-dense extracellular matrix, similar to basement membrane material.

Further Reading

Cervós-Navarro J (1971) Elektronenmikroskopie der Hämangioblastome des ZNS und der angioblastische Meningiome. Acta Neuropathol 19: 184–207

Pēna CE (1975) Intracranial haemangiopericytoma. Ultrastructural evidence of its leiomyoblastic differentiation. Acta Neuropathol 33: 279–284

Popoff NA, Malinn TI, Rosomoff ML (1974) Fine structure of intracranial haemangiopericytoma and angiomatous meningioma. Cancer 34: 1187–1197

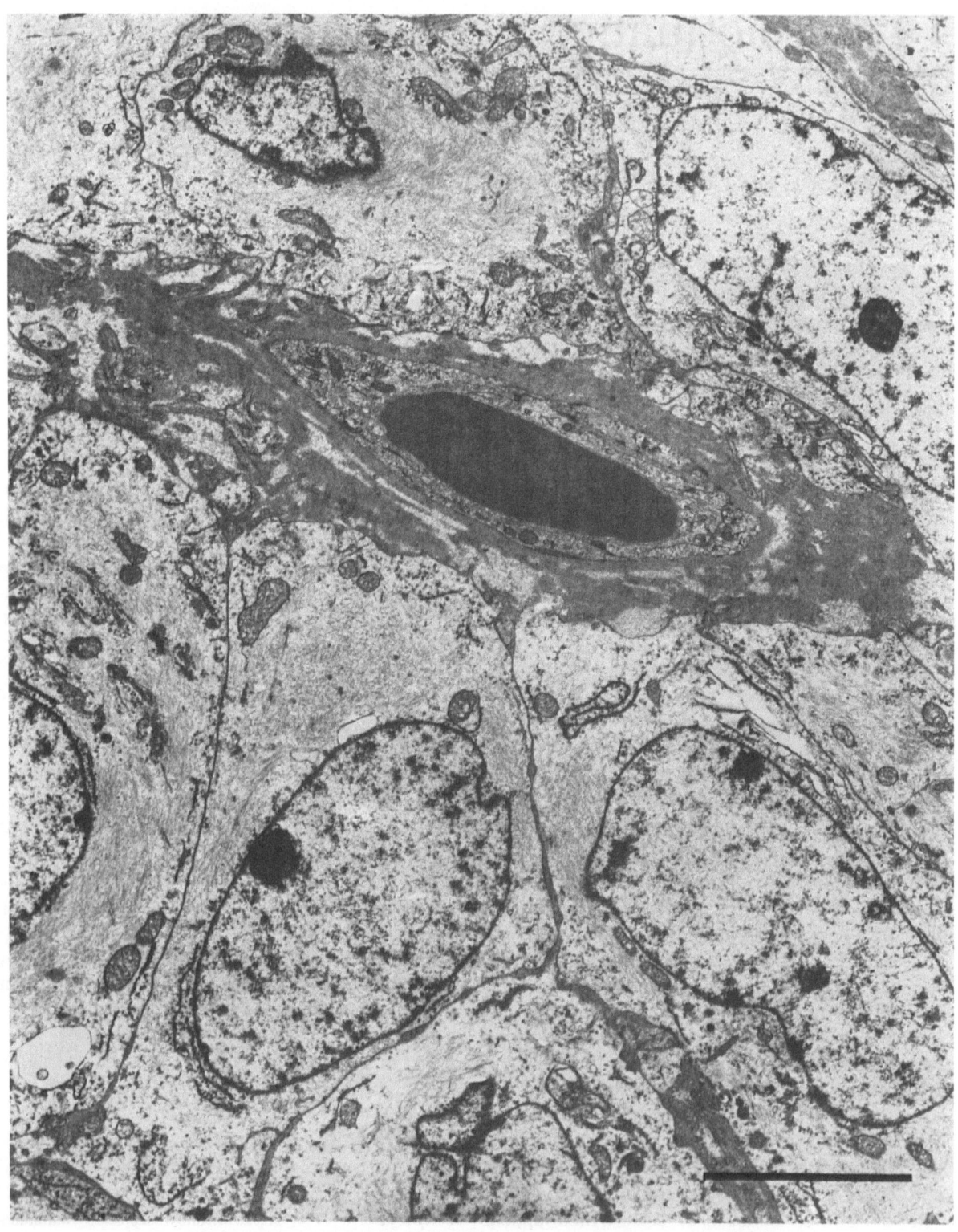

Fig. 14.1. *Angioblastic meningioma.* The tumour cells are typically of uniform, polygonal shape and have rounded, central nuclei. The electron-lucent cytoplasm is usually abundant and filled by 10-nm filaments, as in the cells shown here. Perivascular spaces, like the one in the *centre*, are often wide and filled by electron-dense, amorphous material. The overall appearance is similar to that seen in haemangioblastomas. (Bar = 5 μm)

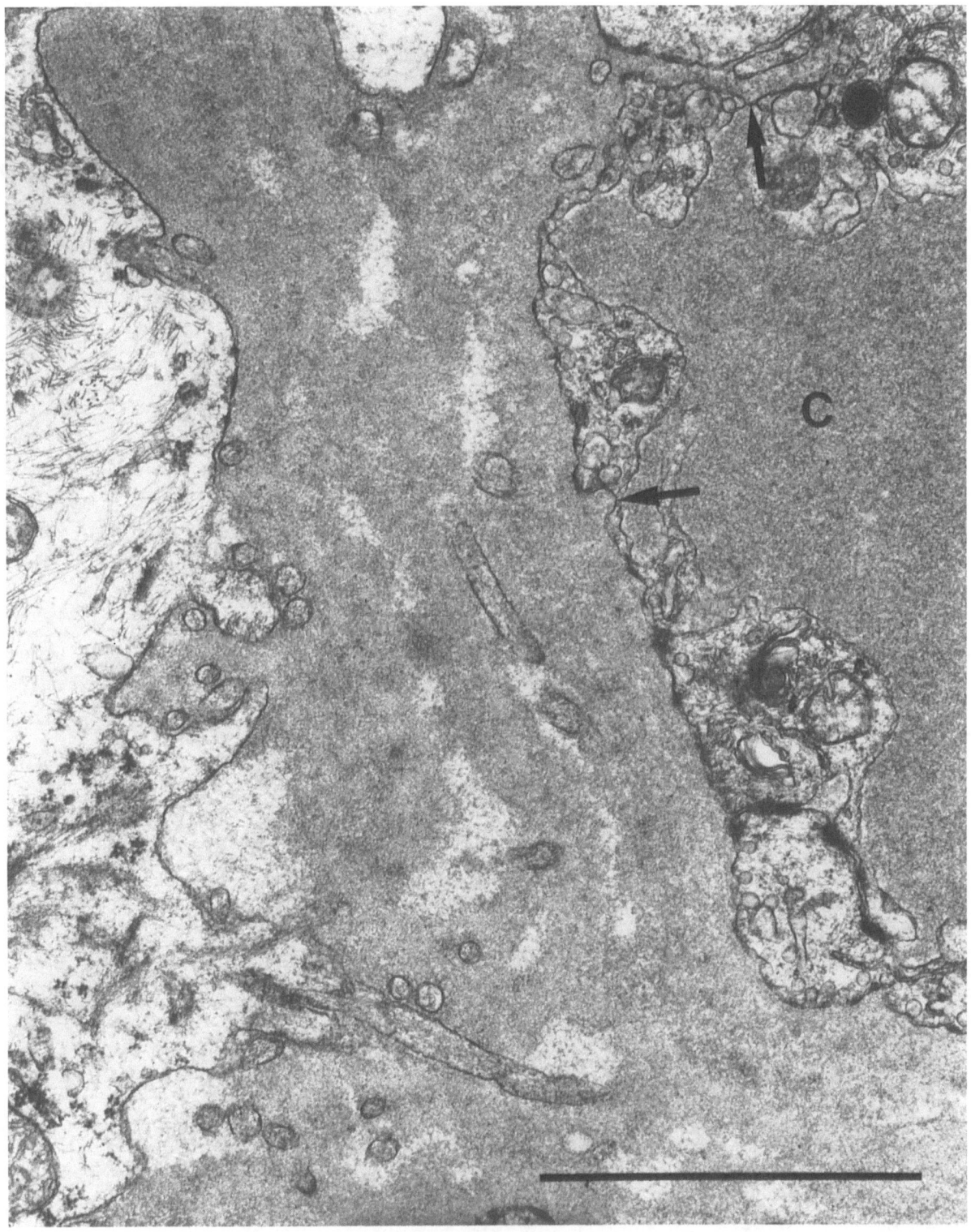

Fig. 14.2. *Angioblastic meningioma.* Numerous thin-walled capillaries are present, like that on the *right* (C). The endothelial lining cells of these capillaries appear morphologically distinct form the tumour cells and are often fenestrated (*arrows*). Amorphous, electron-dense matrix usually fills the perivascular spaces, as can be seen in the *centre* of this field. The tumour cell visible to the *left* of this has typical electron-lucent cytoplasm containing 10-nm filaments. (Bar = 2 μm)

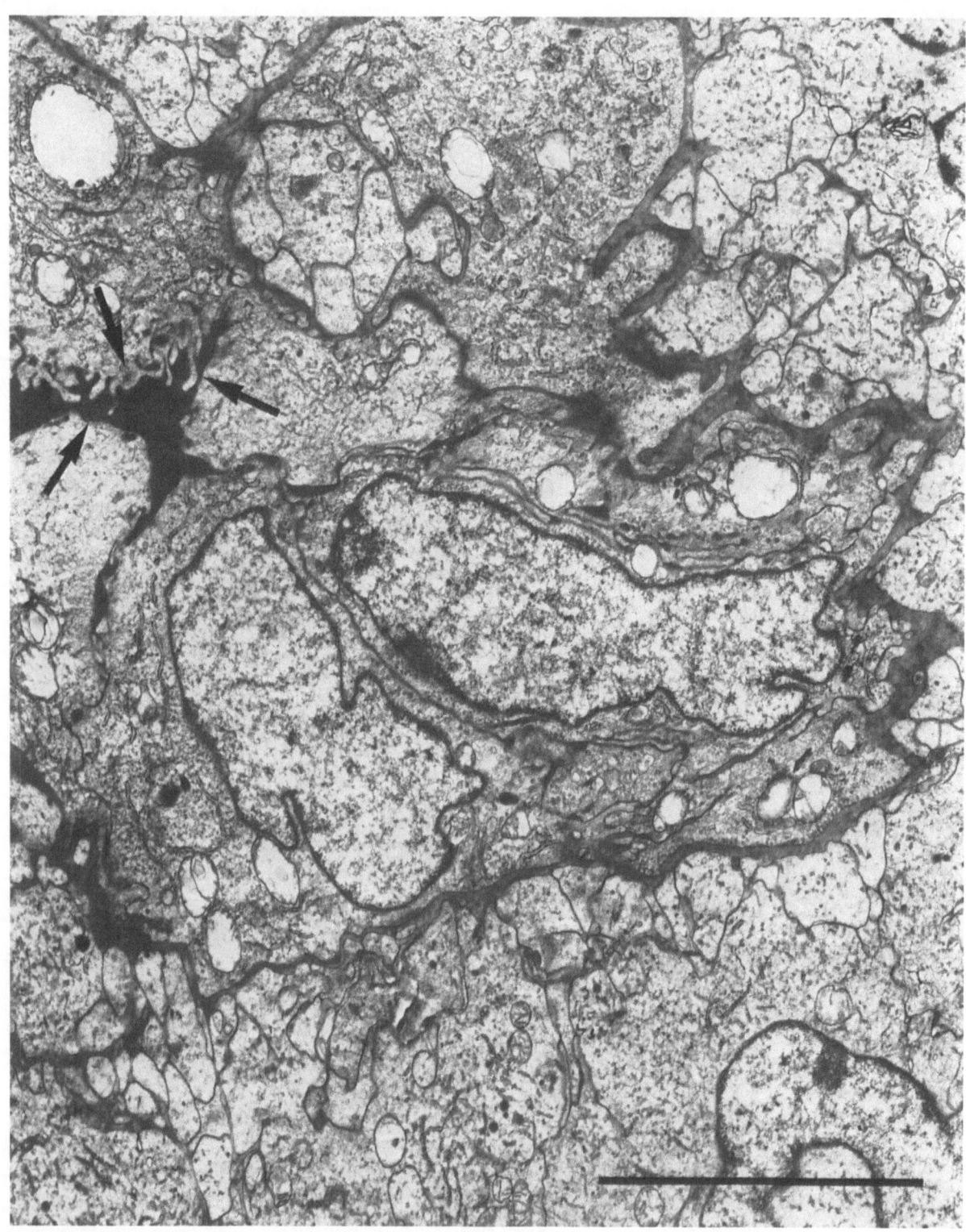

Fig. 14.3. *Haemangiopericytic meningioma.* The tumour cells are often markedly pleomorphic and contain abundant polyribosomes in addition to 10-nm filaments. The numerous abnormal vascular channels have narrow lumina (*arrows*) and are lined by irregular, plump cells similar to the surrounding tumour cells. (Bar = 5 μm)

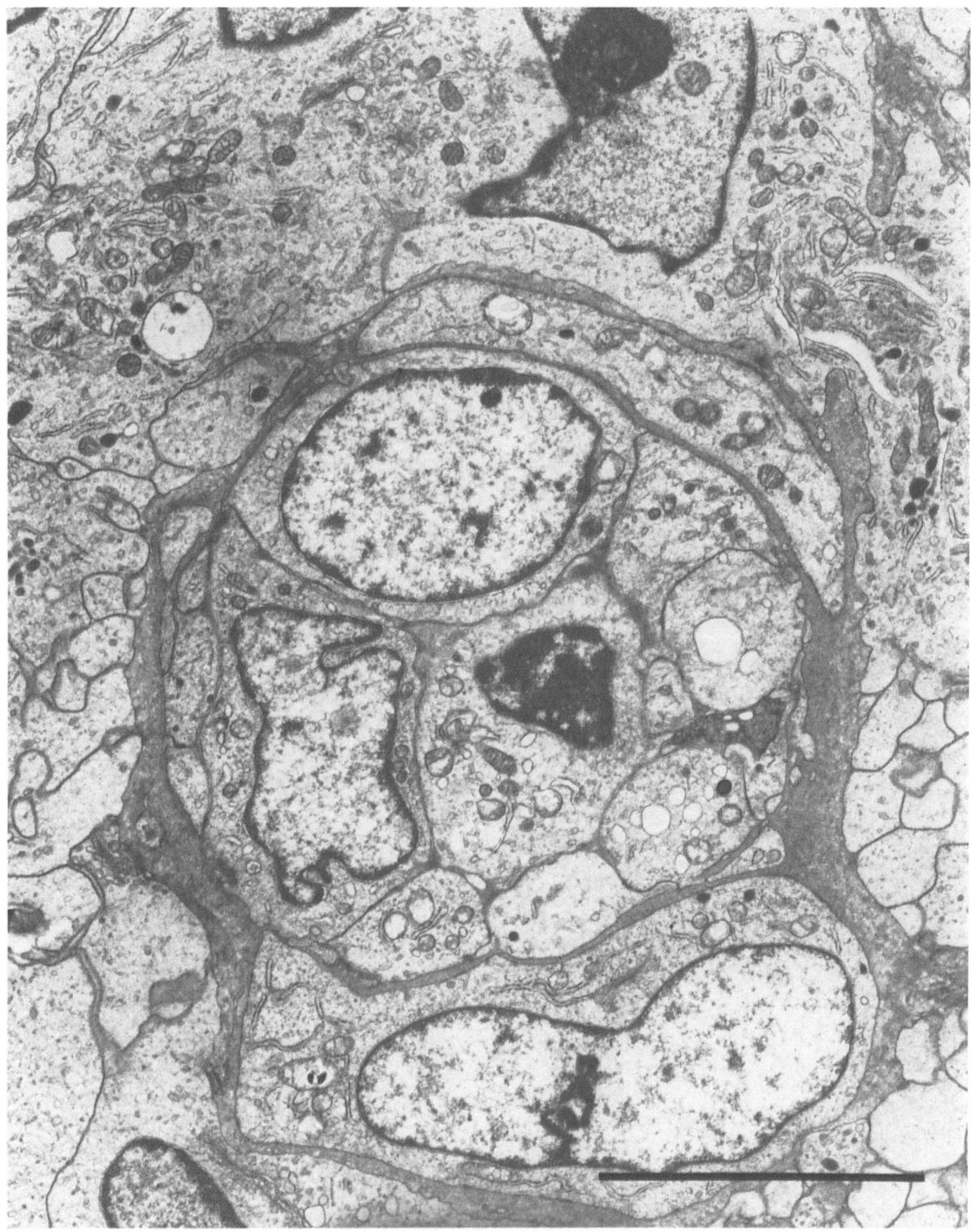

Fig. 14.4. *Haemangiopericytic meningioma.* In some instances, the vascular channels show no detectable endothelial lumina and appear as solid, rounded clumps of cells like that seen in the *centre* of this figure. The clumps are separated from the rest of the tumour only by a thin zone of extracellular space containing electron-dense matrix. (Bar = 5 μm)

15 Schwannoma

The cells of Schwannomas have many ultrastructural features in common with the Schwann cells from which they derive, and show a similar tendency to envelop other structures concentrically. The presence of continuous basement membrane and the absence of pinocytotic vesicles or cell junctions distinguishes the tumour cells from perineurial cells, which may be present in the tumour but do not appear to participate actively in the neoplastic process.

In typical Antoni A areas, the tumour cell bodies are elongate with cigar-shaped nuclei. Their electron-lucent cytoplasm contains 10-nm filaments and they are surrounded by intact basement membranes. They are separated by numerous, parallel fasciculi of tightly packed cell processes, which have an interlocking pattern when cut in cross-section. The processes may be very thin, with virtually no remaining cytoplasm between their plasma membranes, and although basement membrane surrounds each fascicle, it may not extend between tightly apposed individual processes. In some areas, cell processes may form prominent concentric spirals or mesaxon-like structures, reminiscent of primitive myelin sheaths. Axon fibres, however, are not usually present within these tumours.

Antoni B areas differ mainly by virtue of their altered general architecture, and there is no ultrastructural evidence that they are simply the result of tumour degeneration. They may represent areas of increased metabolic activity, and have been reported to show evidence of enhanced fibrin-digesting activity in tissue culture. The cell bodies have an irregular, stellate appearance with ovoid nuclei and numerous cytoplasmic organelles, including lysosomes and membrane-bound dense bodies. There is a loose meshwork of widely separated cell processes, each enclosed by basement membrane. The abundant extracellular space contains redundant basement membrane loops mixed with amorphous and fibrillary material. Together, these constitute the ultrastructural equivalent of reticulin. Both normal collagen fibres (64 nm periodicity) and bundles of long-spaced fibres (up to 150 nm periodicity), called Luse bodies, are also present. Although usually infrequent, typical fibroblasts may be found in most cases and are presumed to be the source of the collagen. There is no definite evidence that the tumour cells themselves participate in collagen production.

Blood vessels have thin, fenestrated, endothelial linings, and the hyaline thickening seen on light microscopy consists ultrastructurally of surrounding concentric lamellae of collagen and reduplicated basement membrane. The adjacent perivascular tumour tissue may appear degenerate, with lipid-laden cells and disrupted plasma membranes. These changes are possibly the result of local hypoxia caused by the blood vessel wall alterations.

Further Reading

Cravioto H (1969) The ultrastructure of acoustic nerve tumours. Acta Neuropathol 12: 116–140

Erlandson RA, Woodruff JM (1982) Peripheral nerve sheath tumours: an electron microscopic study of 43 cases. Cancer 49: 273–287

Luse SA (1960) Electron microscopic studies of brain tumours. Neurology 10: 881–905

Sian CS, Ryan SF (1981) The ultrastructure of neurilemoma with emphasis on Antoni B tissue. Hum Pathol 12: 145–160

Waggener JD (1966) Ultrastructure of benign peripheral nerve sheath tumours. Cancer 19: 699–709

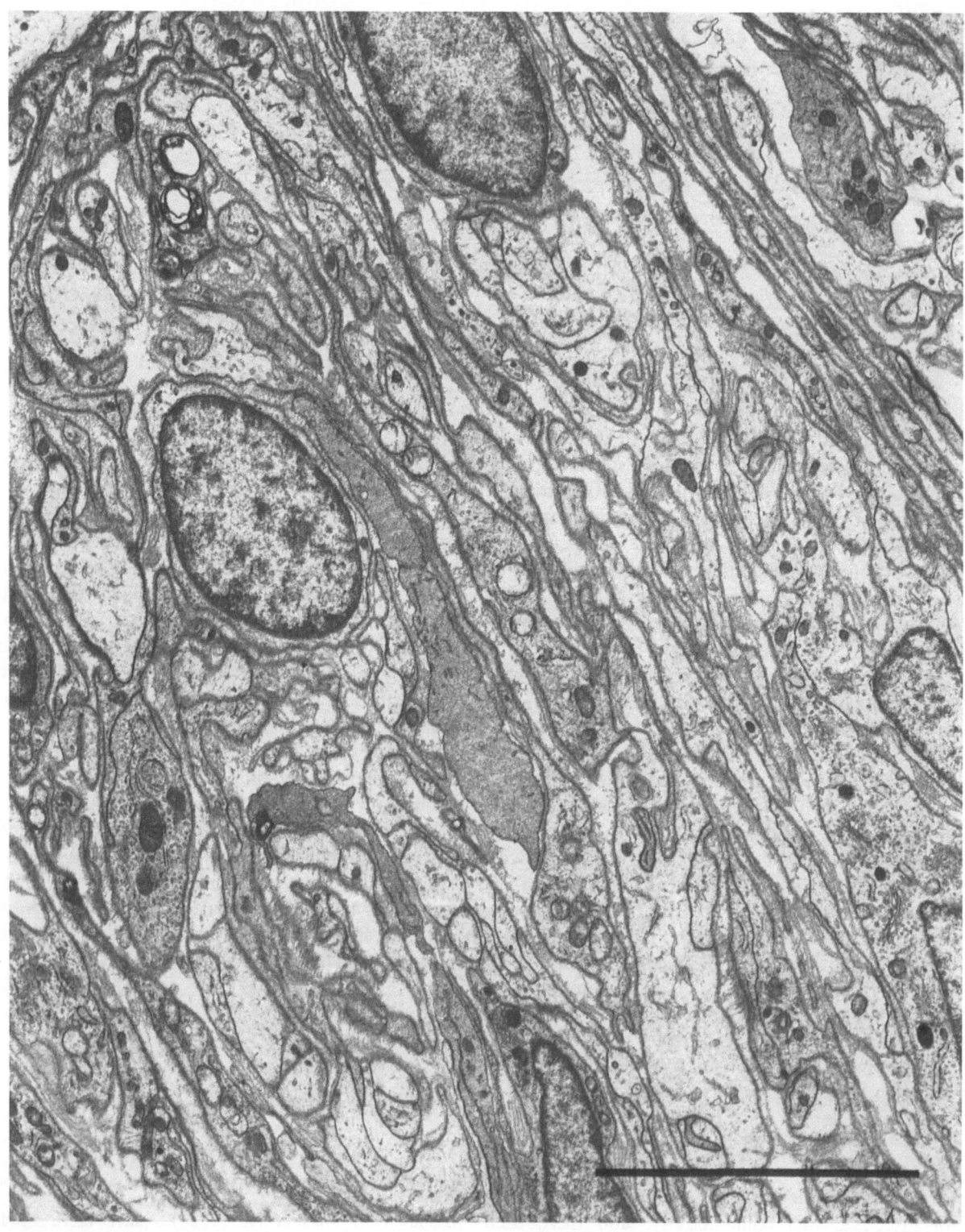

Fig. 15.1. *Schwannoma.* In Antoni A areas, the cell bodies are elongate and separated by numerous, parallel bundles of electron-lucent processes. These show an interlocking pattern when viewed in cross-section, as in the *lower left* of this figure. In contrast to Antoni B areas, the cell processes are usually closely packed together, with little intervening extracellular space. (Bar = 5 μm)

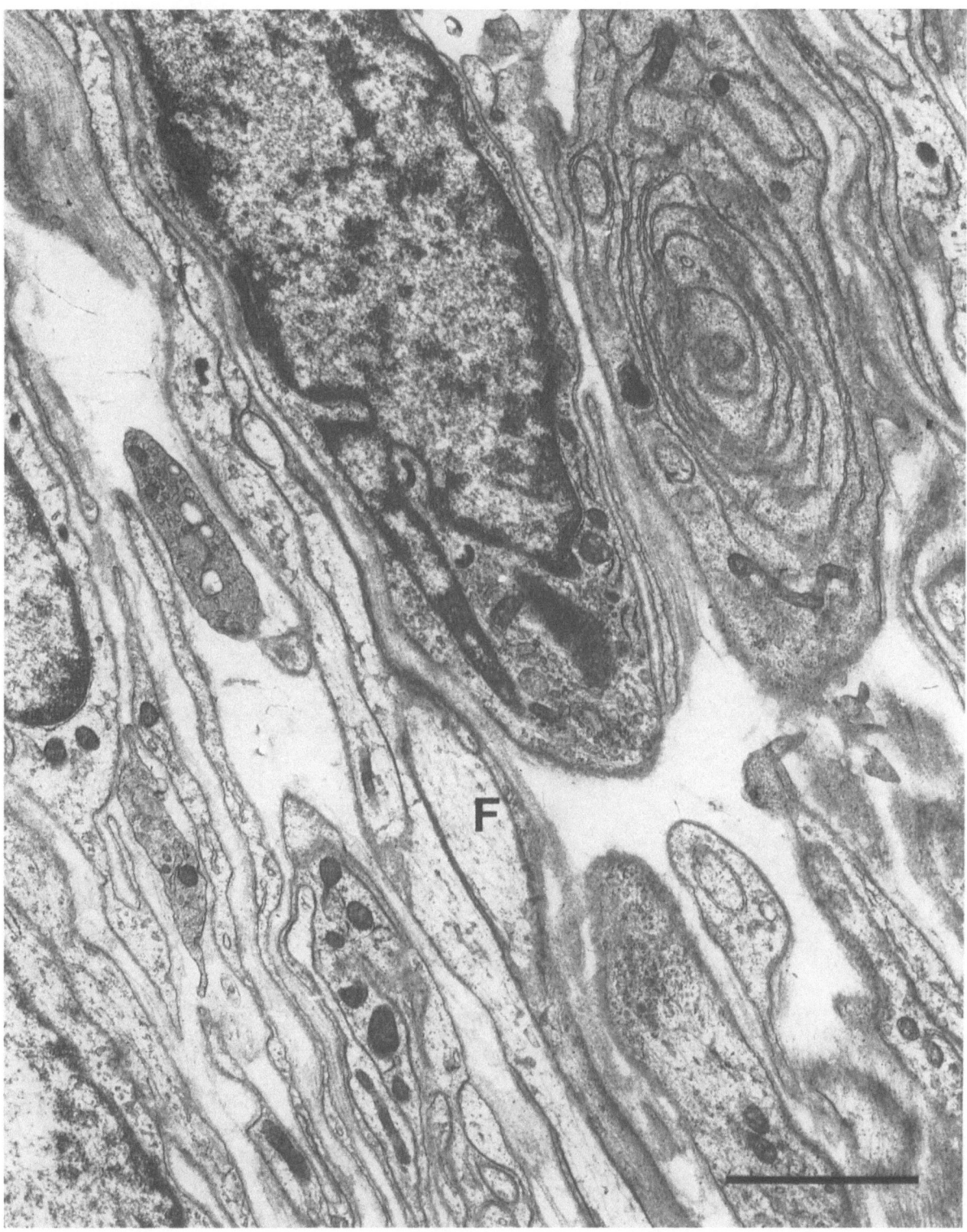

Fig. 15.2. *Schwannoma.* The tumour cell processes contain 10-nm filaments (*F*) and may occasionally form concentric spirals reminiscent of primitive myelin sheaths, like that seen in the *top right corner*. In Antoni A areas, the processes are often very thin, as seen at the *bottom left*, and have little remaining cytoplasm separating their plasma membranes. Basement membrane surrounds both the processes and cell bodies but may not extend between individual, tightly apposed processes. (Bar = 2 μm)

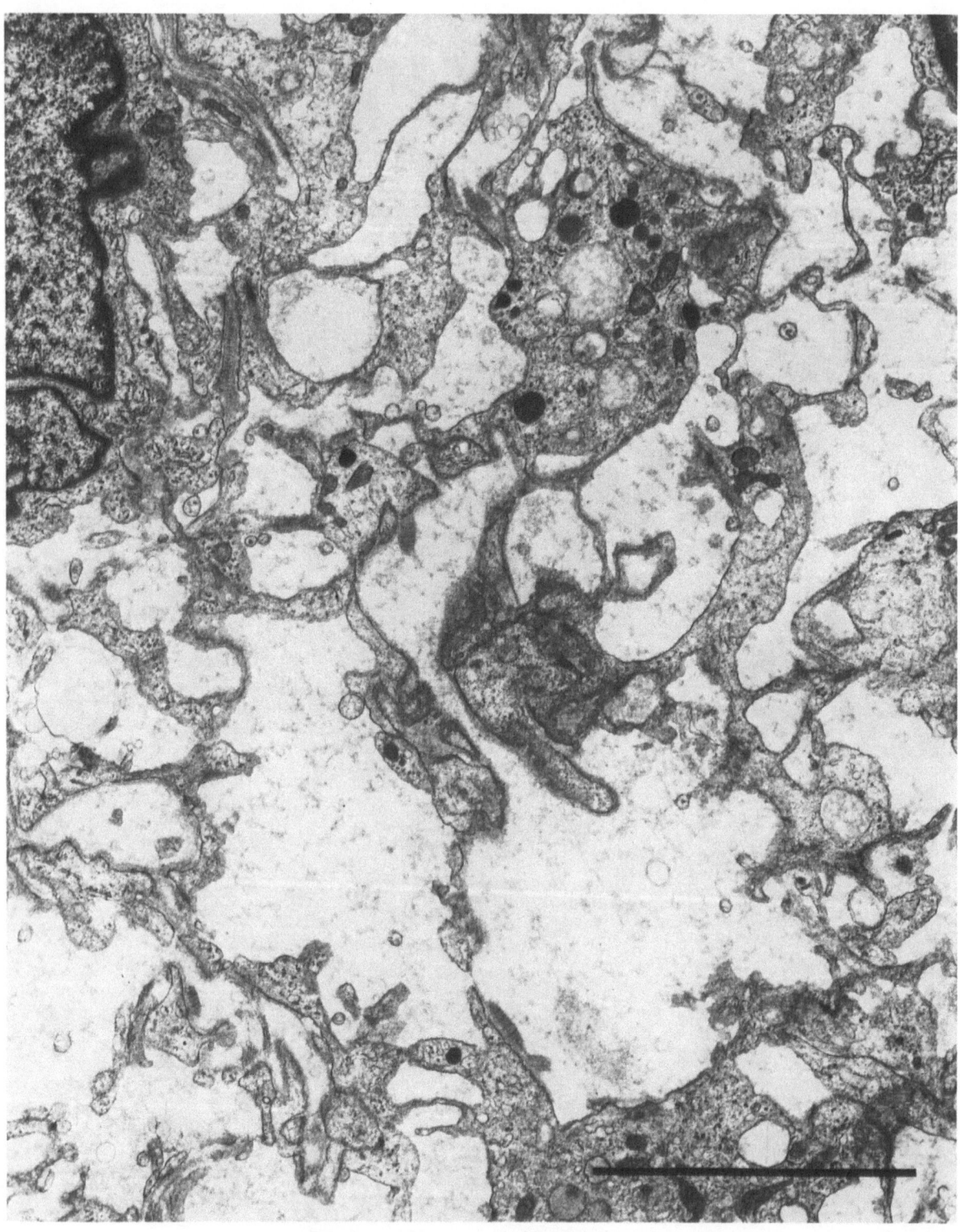

Fig. 15.3. *Schwannoma.* Antoni B areas do not usually appear degenerate but have an altered general architecture, as shown in this figure. The cell bodies have an irregular, stellate shape and their processes are widely separated to form a loose mesh. The cell cytoplasm often contains increased organelles, including lysosomal vacuoles and membrane-bound dense bodies. (Bar = 5 μm)

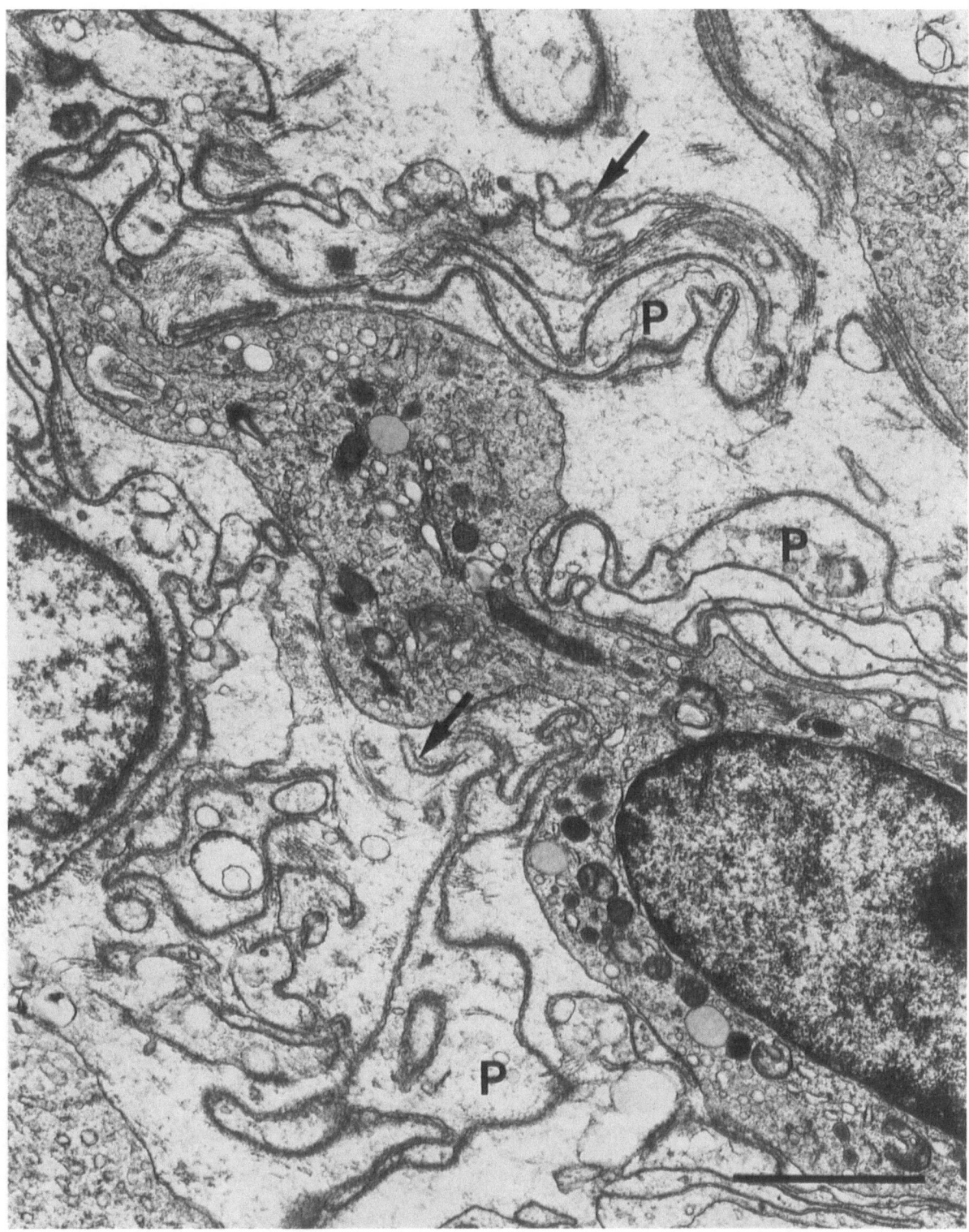

Fig. 15.4. *Schwannoma.* In Antoni B areas, the tumour cell processes (*P*) are individually enclosed by basement membrane, which may form redundant loops (*arrows*). Occasional cells, like that in the *centre*, have electron-dense cytoplasm containing numerous pinocytotic vesicles and are not surrounded by basement membrane. (Bar = 2 µm)

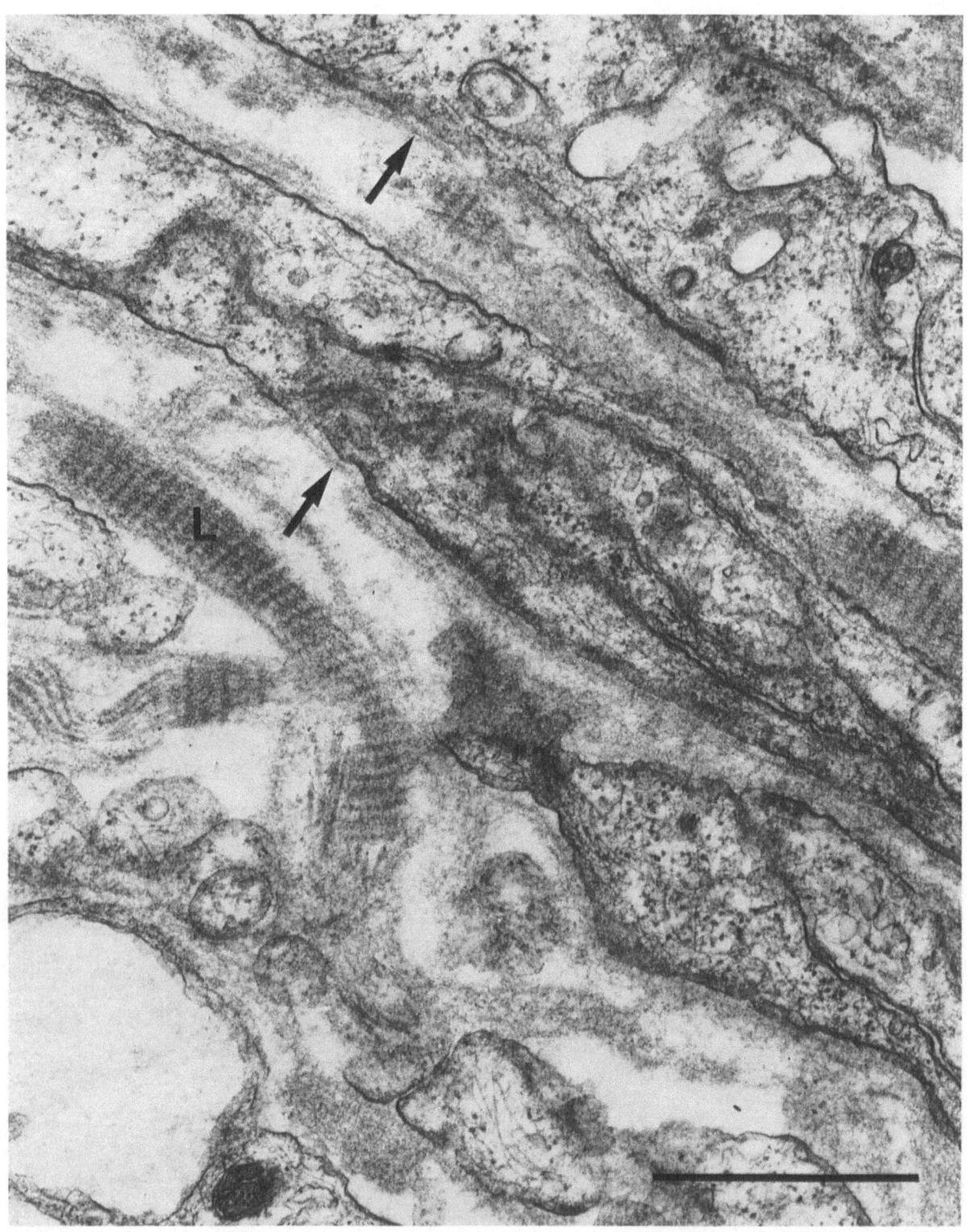

Fig. 15.5. *Schwannoma.* The extracellular space in Antoni B areas contains both normal collagen (64 nm periodicity) and bundles of long-spaced collagen fibres (up to 150 nm periodicity). These bundles have a distinctive banded appearance and are called Luse bodies (*L*). The basement membranes (*arrows*) and associated amorphous material in the extracellular space are the ultrastructural equivalent of reticulin. (Bar = 1 μm)

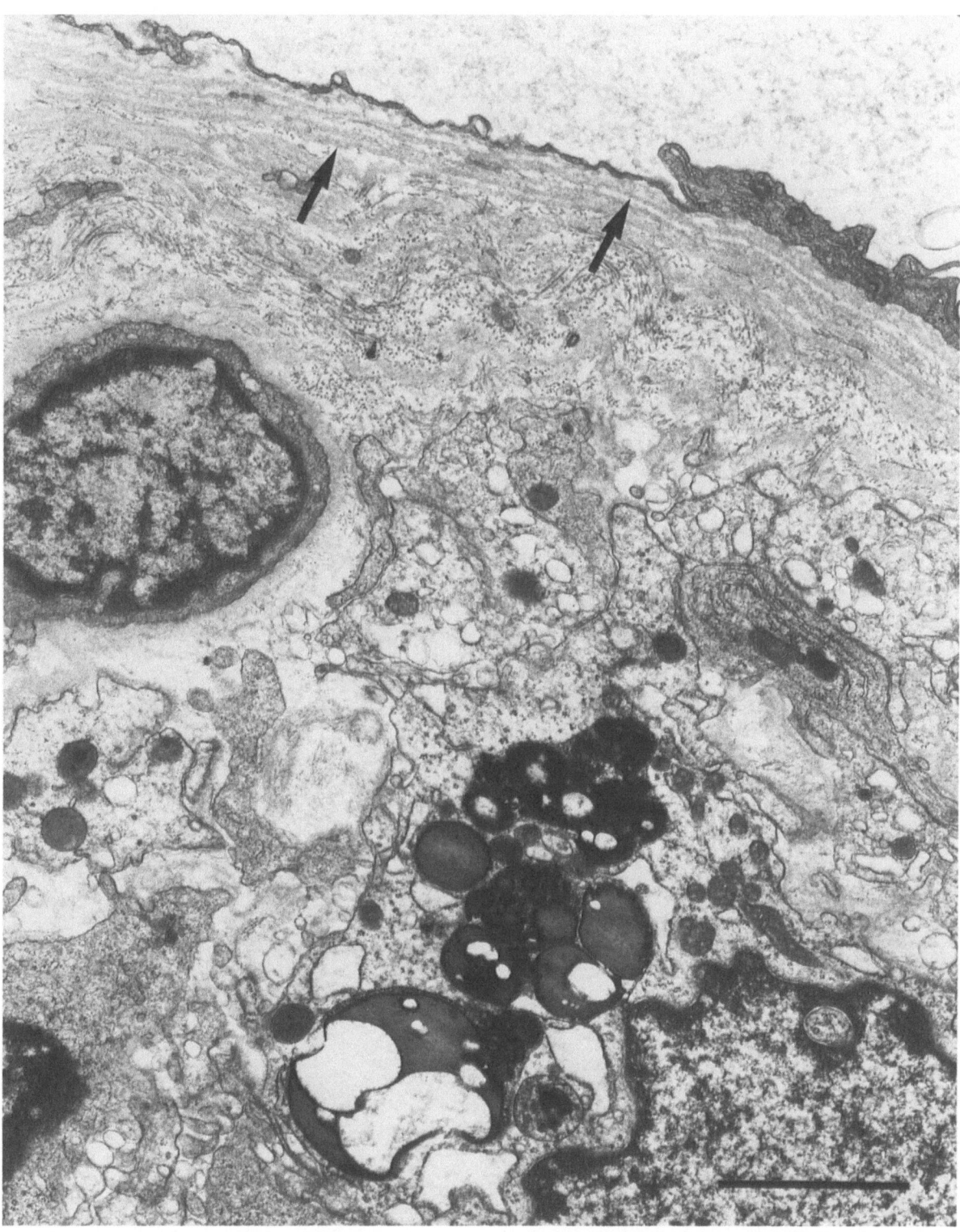

Fig. 15.6. *Schwannoma.* Capillary vessels have a thin, fenestrated, endothelial lining, like that seen at the *top* of this figure, but they are often enveloped by concentric lamellae of collagen and reduplicated basement membranes (*arrows*). This results in the characteristic hyaline thickening of vessel walls seen on light microscopy. The surrounding tumour tissue frequently appears degenerate, as in this case, with lipid-laden phagocytes and vacuolated tumour cell cytoplasm. (Bar = 2 μm)

16 Neurofibroma

Neurofibromas are fundamentally tumours of Schwann cells, and although fibroblastic cells are always present, the predominant type of tumour cell is ultrastructurally similar to a neoplastic Schwann cell. These cells are of very variable size and shape, with numerous, irregular cytoplasmic processes and irregular nuclear outlines. Their perikaryal cytoplasm contains varied organelles, including abundant polyribosomes, and is surrounded by an intact basement membrane. The cell bodies and their processes are widely separated by a greatly expanded extracellular space, which is a characteristic ultrastructural feature of these tumours and contains amorphous or fibrillary material mixed with abundant collagen fibres. The collagen may have an abnormally long periodicity and form Luse bodies (see Chap. 15). The processes of these tumour cells have electron-lucent cytoplasm filled with 10-nm filaments and, like the cell bodies, are surrounded by basement membrane. This often forms proliferated or redundant loops in the extracellular space. Although irregularly arranged, the cell processes sometimes interdigitate and can resemble those found in Schwannomas. Like true Schwann cell processes, they often encircle bundles of collagen fibres to form "collagen pockets" and may also envelop the small bundles of axons which are usually found running through the tumour. These axons are sometimes thinly myelinated and probably originate from pre-existing nerve fascicles, which have been enveloped by tumour but still retain perineurial sheaths. Individual axons have been observed traversing the sheaths of such nerve fascicles and entering the extracellular space of the tumour.

The second main cell type within these tumours resembles a fibroblast and may not be actively involved in the neoplastic process. Although a much more prominent feature than the fibroblasts seen in Schwannomas, the fibroblastic cells present in neurofibromas are less common than the Schwann cell type. They have an irregular, flattened shape with thin terminal processes and cytoplasm which often contains abundant cisternae of rough endoplasmic reticulum. There is no surrounding basement membrane and the plasma membranes are often intimately associated with the abundant extracellular collagen.

In summary, the main differences of these tumours from Schwannomas at ultrastructural level are the greatly expanded extracellular space, which often contains bundles of thinly myelinated or unmyelinated axons, the large amounts of extracellular collagen, and the consistent presence of both Schwann cell and fibroblastic cell types.

Further Reading

Erlandson RA, Woodruff JM (1982) Peripheral nerve sheath tumours: an electron microscopic study of 43 cases. Cancer 49: 273–287

Lassmann H, Jurecka W, Lassmann G, Gebhart W, Matrash H, Watzek G (1977) Different types of benign nerve sheath tumours. Light microscopy, electron microscopy and autoradiography. Virchows Arch [A] 375: 197–210

Poirier J, Escourelle R, Castaigne P (1968) Les neurofibromas de la malodie de Recklinghausen. Étude ultrastructurale et place neurologique par rapport aux neurinomes. Acta Neuropathol 10: 279–294

Waggener JD (1966) Ultrastructure of benign peripheral nerve sheath tumours. Cancer 19: 699–709

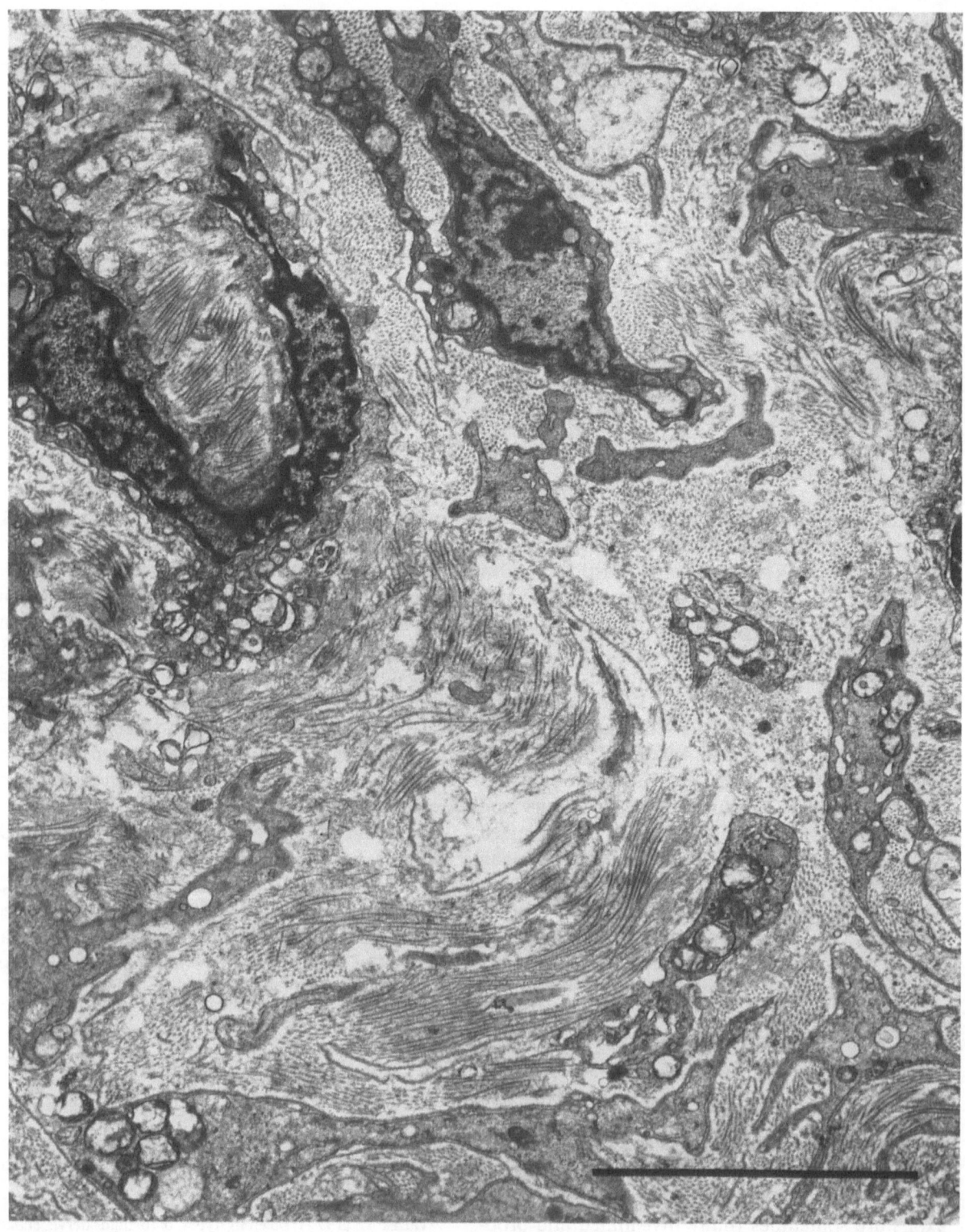

Fig. 16.1. *Neurofibroma.* A prominent ultrastructural feature of these tumours is the greatly expanded extracellular space. As can be seen here, this usually contains abundant collagen, together with the widely separated tumour cell bodies and their irregular processes. (Bar = 5 μm)

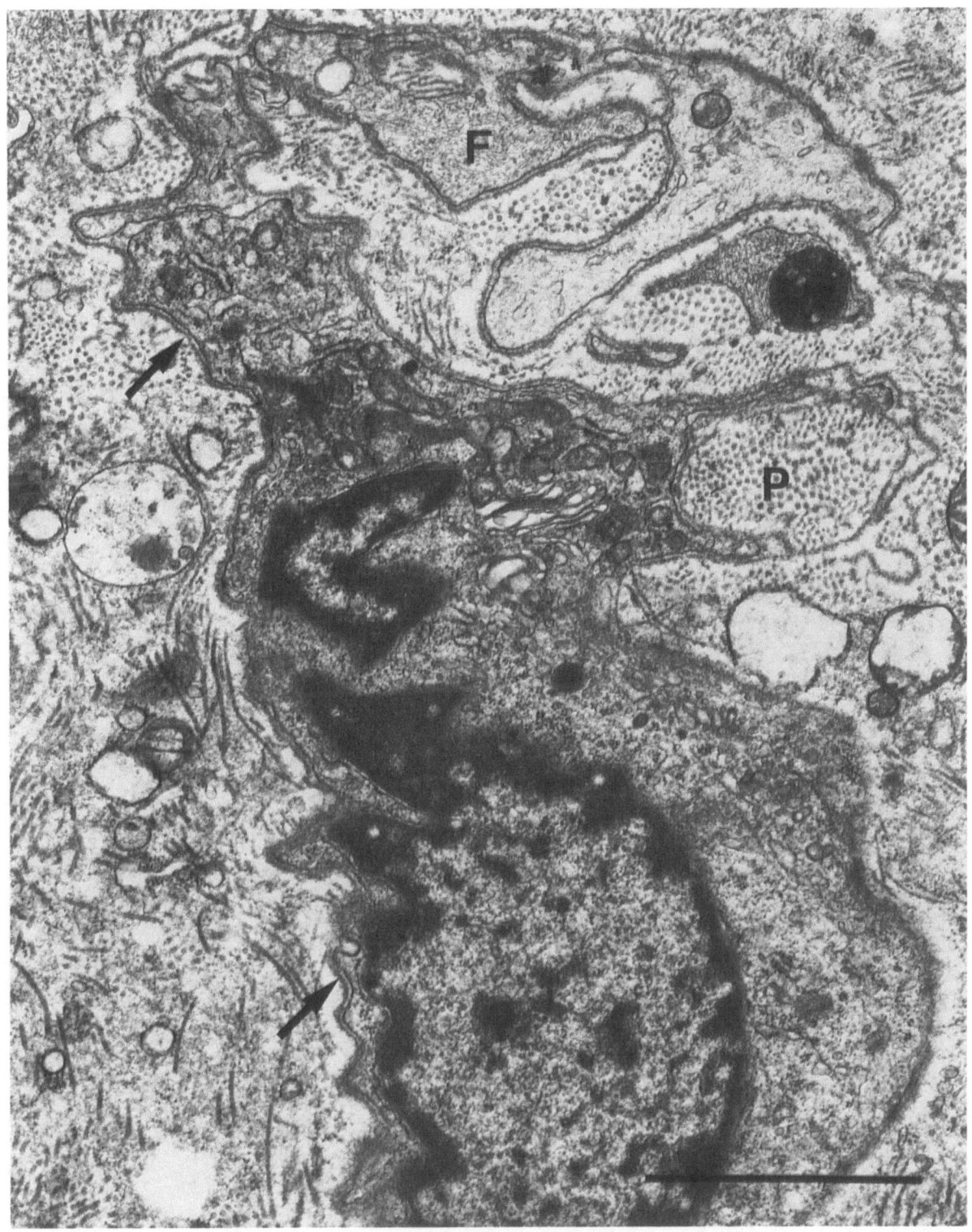

Fig. 16.2. *Neurofibroma.* The principal cell type of these tumours is illustrated here and resembles a neoplastic Schwann cell. The cell bodies are irregularly rounded in shape and enveloped by intact basement membrane (*arrows*). The processes of these cells, visible at the *top* of this figure, have electron-lucent cytoplasm filled with 10-nm filaments (*F*) and are again surrounded by basement membranes. The cell cytoplasm and basement membrane may sometimes enclose collagen pockets (*P*). (Bar = 2 μm)

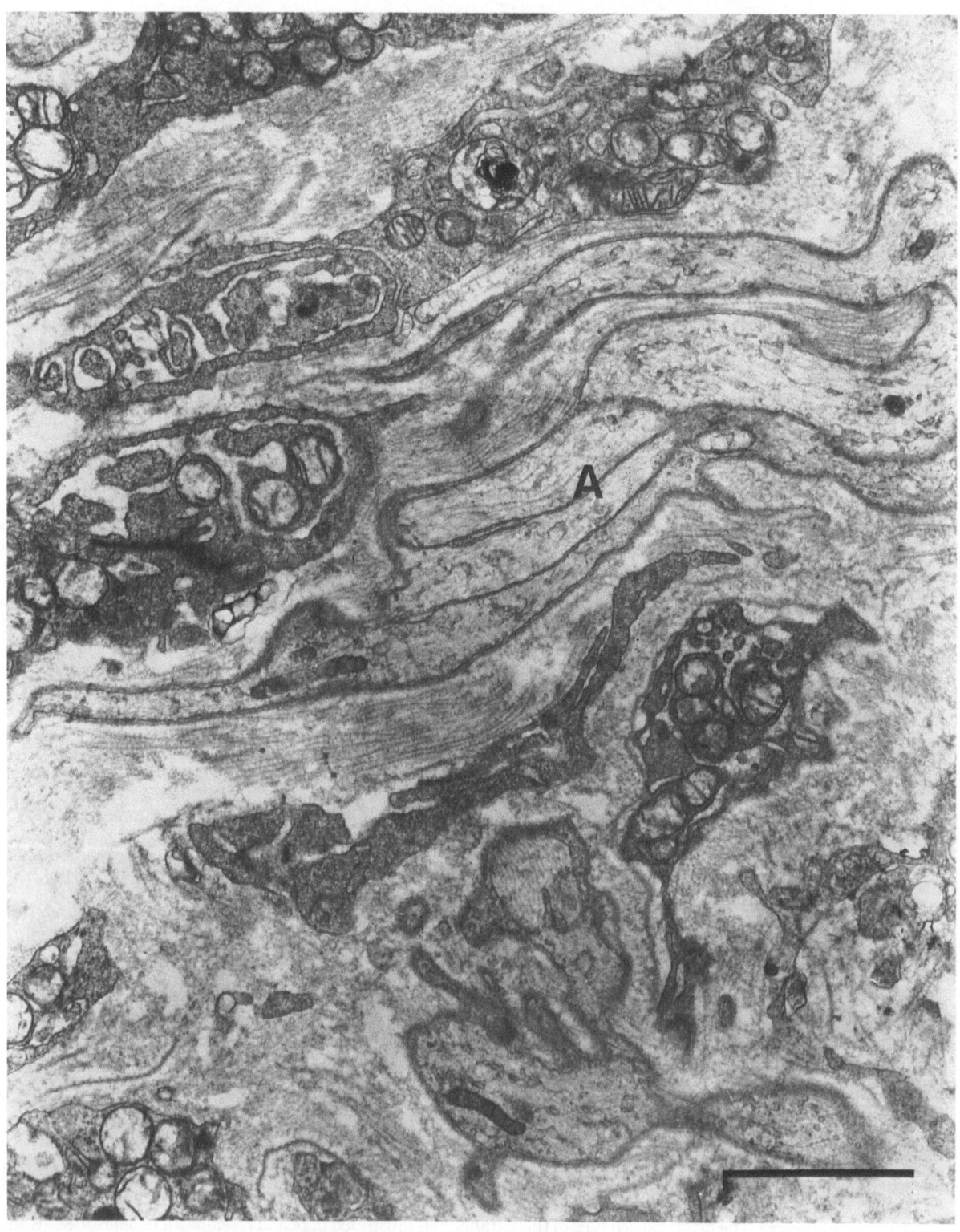

Fig. 16.3. *Neurofibroma.* Small bundles of axons (*A*) often traverse the extracellular space, as seen in the field shown here. These axons are often enveloped by Schwann cell-like neoplastic processes and can be thinly myelinated in some cases. (Bar = 2 μm)

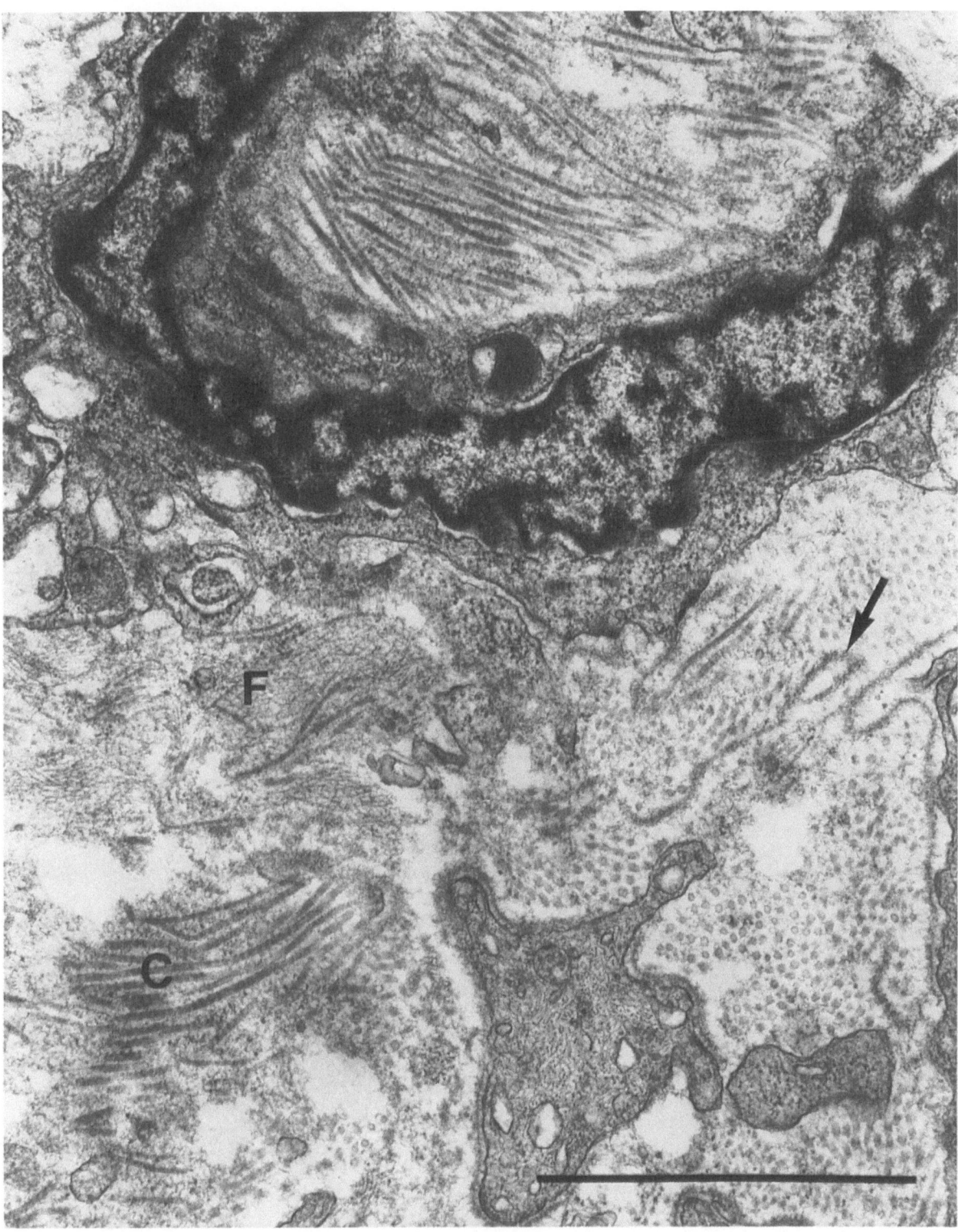

Fig. 16.4. *Neurofibroma.* The extracellular space contains filamentous or amorphous material (*F*) and redundant basement membrane loops (*arrow*) in addition to the abundant collagen fibres (*C*). An irregular, flattened, fibroblastic type of tumour cell is present at the *top* of this figure. Although a consistent feature, these cells are less common than the Schwann cell type and lack basement membrane. They are often intimately associated with the extracellular collagen and may be responsible for its production. (Bar = 2 μm)

17 Haemangioblastoma

Haemangioblastomas are ultrastructurally very similar to some forms of angioblastic meningioma, but the precise relationship between these two tumours is uncertain, and the nature of the cells from which haemangioblastomas originate is still controversial. Three different cell types can normally be distinguished in these tumours, but it is not clear whether all of these are actively involved in the neoplastic process.

In most cases, sheets of intervascular stromal cells are the predominant component of the tumour. These cells have uniform, large, rounded nuclei and abundant, electron-lucent cytoplasm which forms blunt peripheral processes. Nuclear chromatin is usually evenly dispersed and there may be prominent nucleoli. Cytoplasmic organelles are generally rather sparse, but 7-nm filaments are typically abundant and concentric whorls of rough endoplasmic reticulum may be a prominent feature in some places. Many of these cells also contain large lipid droplets or empty, non-membrane-bound vacuoles. In some cases, very occasional pinocytotic vesicles and patchy, incomplete basement membranes may be found, but unlike the endothelial cells present, the stromal cells do not form junctional attachments. Stromal cells are often separated by abundant extracellular space which contains amorphous ground substance, scanty collagen fibres and occasional mast cells with their typical electron-dense cytoplasmic granules.

The other two main cell types are the endothelial cells and pericytes, which form numerous capillary channels of essentially normal structure. The endothelial cells have flattened, irregular nuclei and electron-dense cytoplasm containing 7-nm filaments and numerous pinocytotic vesicles. They show occasional fenestrations and are joined together in a single, thin layer by elongate desmosomes. They are surrounded by an intact basement membrane, and outside this the pericytes are loosely arranged, separated from the stromal cells by a second, outer basement membrane. The pericytes closely resemble the endothelial cells, but are not linked together by desmosome junctions.

Although the stromal cells usually appear morphologically distinct from the endothelial cells and pericytes, a spectrum of ultrastructural appearances can be observed in some tumours. Moreover, in tissue culture experiments, typical stromal cells may acquire more prominent endothelial characteristics, including numerous pinocytotic vesicles and intact basement membranes. Such observations suggest that haemangioblastomas are most likely to be vasoformative tumours of a single basic cell type, which probably has a common developmental origin with both endothelial cells and pericytes.

Further Reading

Castaigne P, David M, Petuiset B, Escourolle R, Poirier J (1968) L'Ultrastructure des hémangioblastomes du système nerveux central. Rev Neurol 118: 5–26

Cervós-Navarro J (1971) Elektronenmikroskopie der Hämangioblastome des ZNS und der angioblastischen Meningiome. Acta Neuropathol 19: 184–207

Kawamura J, Garcia JH, Kamijo Y (1973) Cerebellar haemangioblastoma: histogenesis of stromal cells. Cancer 31: 1528–1540

Spence AM, Rubinstein LJ (1975) Cerebellar capillary haemangioblastoma: its histogenesis studied by organ culture and electron microscopy. Cancer 35: 326–341

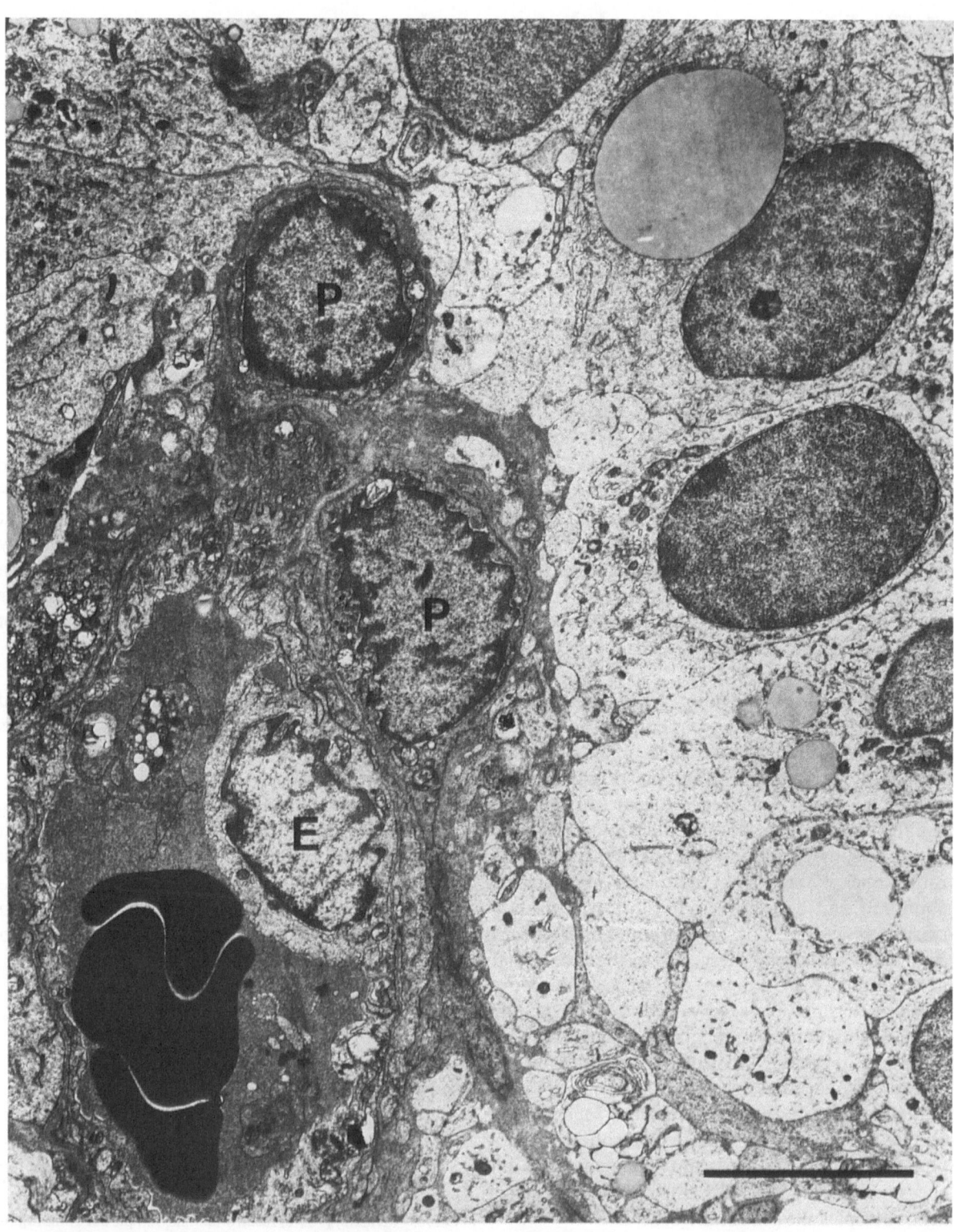

Fig. 17.1. *Haemangioblastoma.* Three separate cell types can normally be distinguished. The intervascular stromal cells, visible on the *right*, have uniform rounded nuclei and abundant, electron-lucent cytoplasm. They often contain large lipid droplets or empty vacuoles, as in many of the cells here. The endothelial cells (*E*) and surrounding pericytes (*P*) form numerous capillary channels of essentially normal architecture, like the one present on the *left*. (Bar = 5 μm)

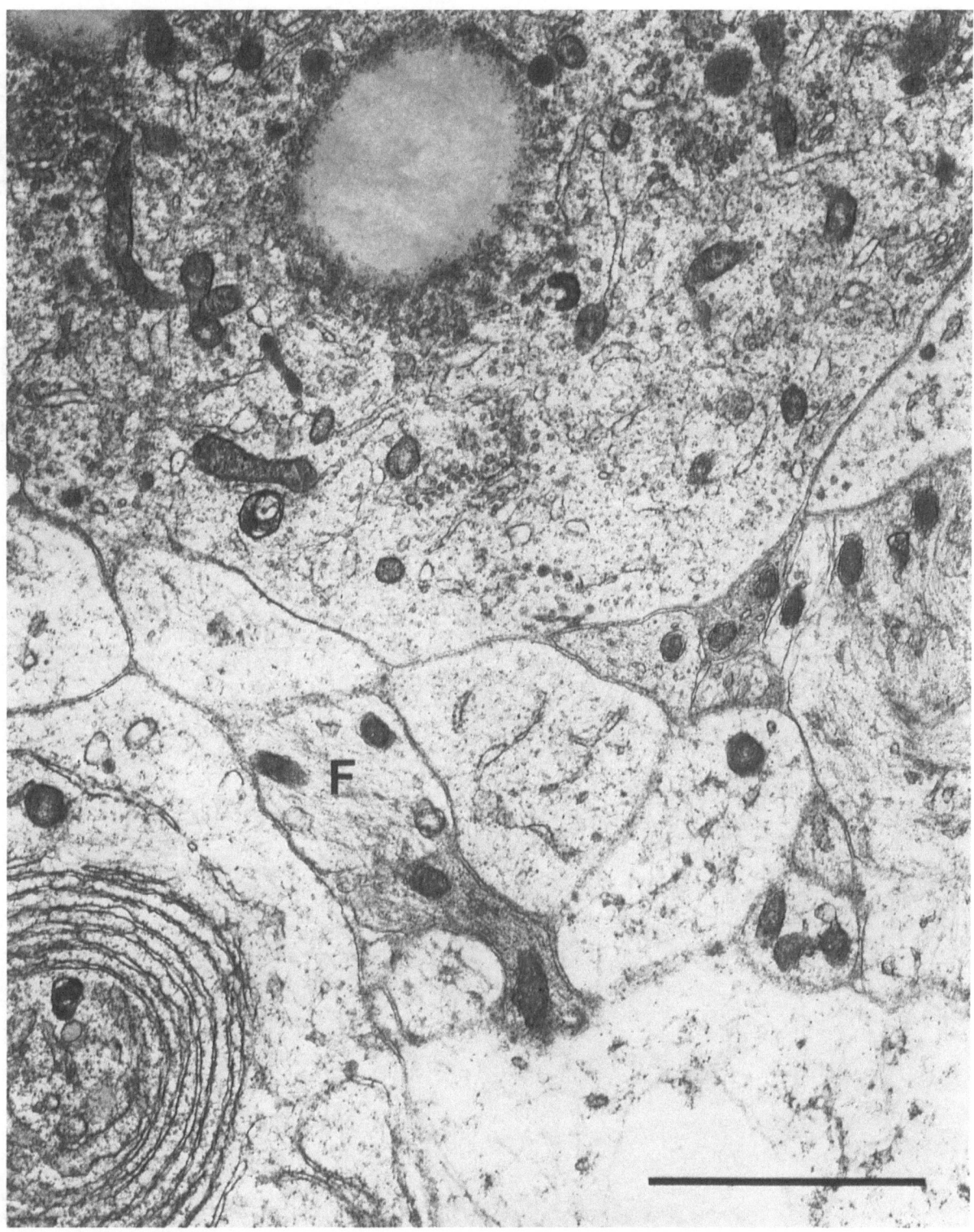

Fig. 17.2. *Haemangioblastoma.* The cytoplasm of the stromal cells contains abundant 7-nm filaments (*F*). Prominent whorls of rough endoplasmic reticulum may also be present, as in the *lower left corner*. Lipid vacuoles, like the one in the uppermost cell here, are not membrane bound. There are no junctions between adjacent cells. (Bar = 2 μm)

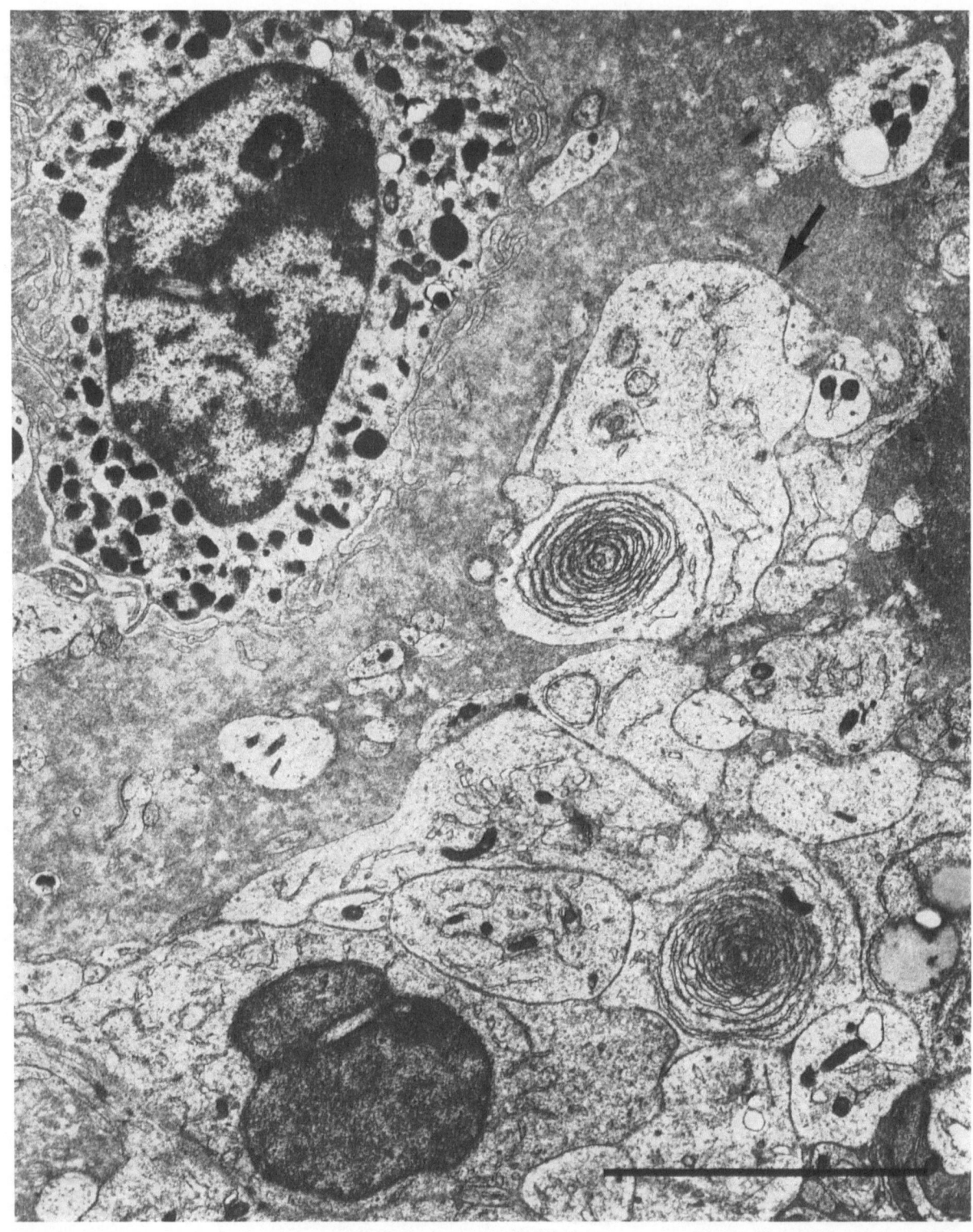

Fig. 17.3. *Haemangioblastoma.* The extracellular space, which can be seen in the *upper part* of this figure, is filled by amorphous matrix and may be very extensive in some areas. Scattered mast cells may be present, like the one seen at the *top* here, and contain characteristic, electron-dense cytoplasmic granules. Some stromal cells may be surrounded by patchy basement membrane (*arrow*), although it is entirely lacking in most cases. Two of the stromal cells in this field contain characteristic whorls of rough endoplasmic reticulum. (Bar = 5 μm)

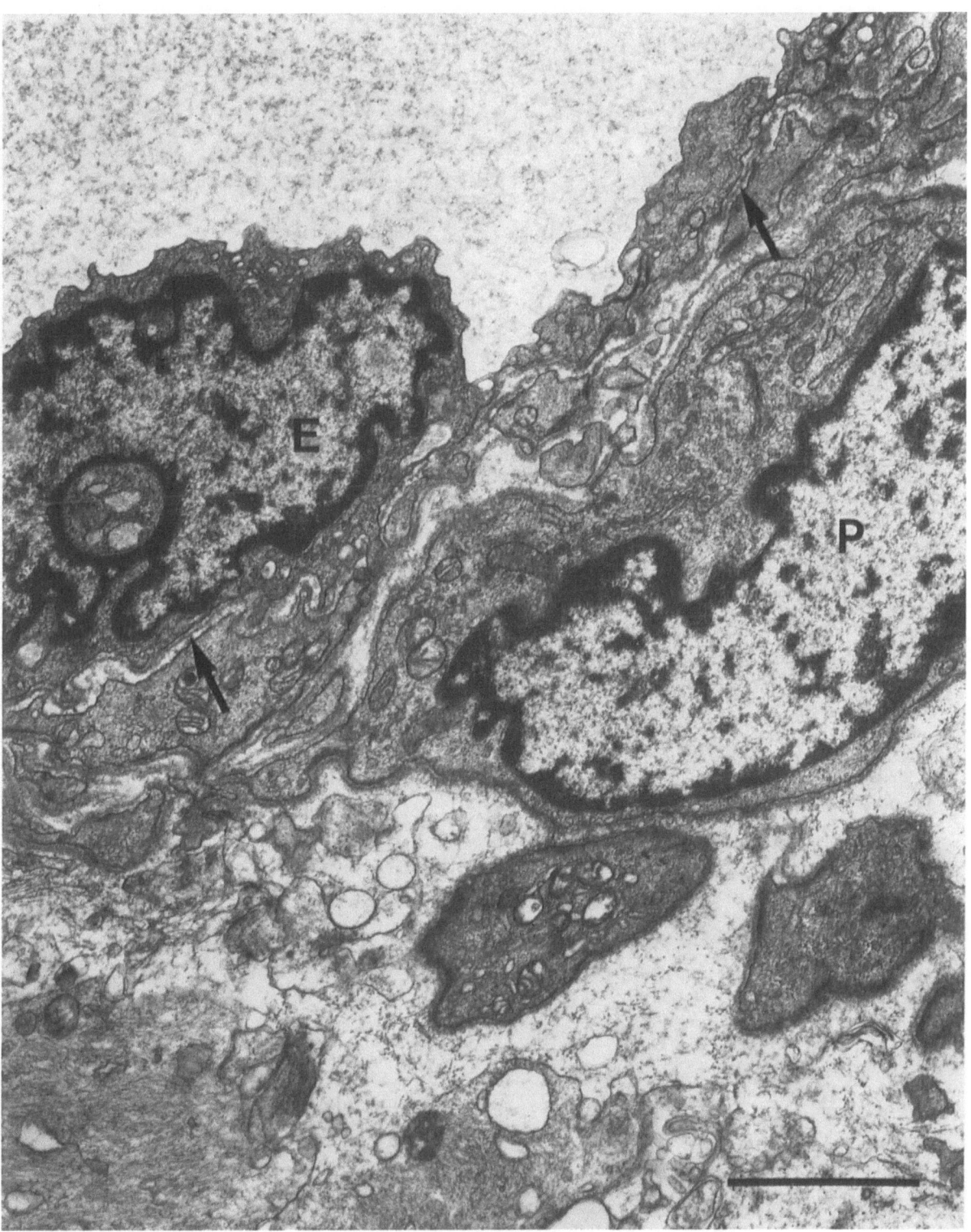

Fig. 17.4. *Haemangioblastoma.* The capillary endothelial cells (*E*) have irregular, flattened nuclei and form a single, thin layer around the vascular lumen, visible at the *top* of this figure. The endothelial cells are surrounded by intact basement membrane (*arrows*), and pericytes (*P*) of similar morphology lie outside this. The pericytes are enclosed by a second, outer basement membrane. (Bar = 2 μm)

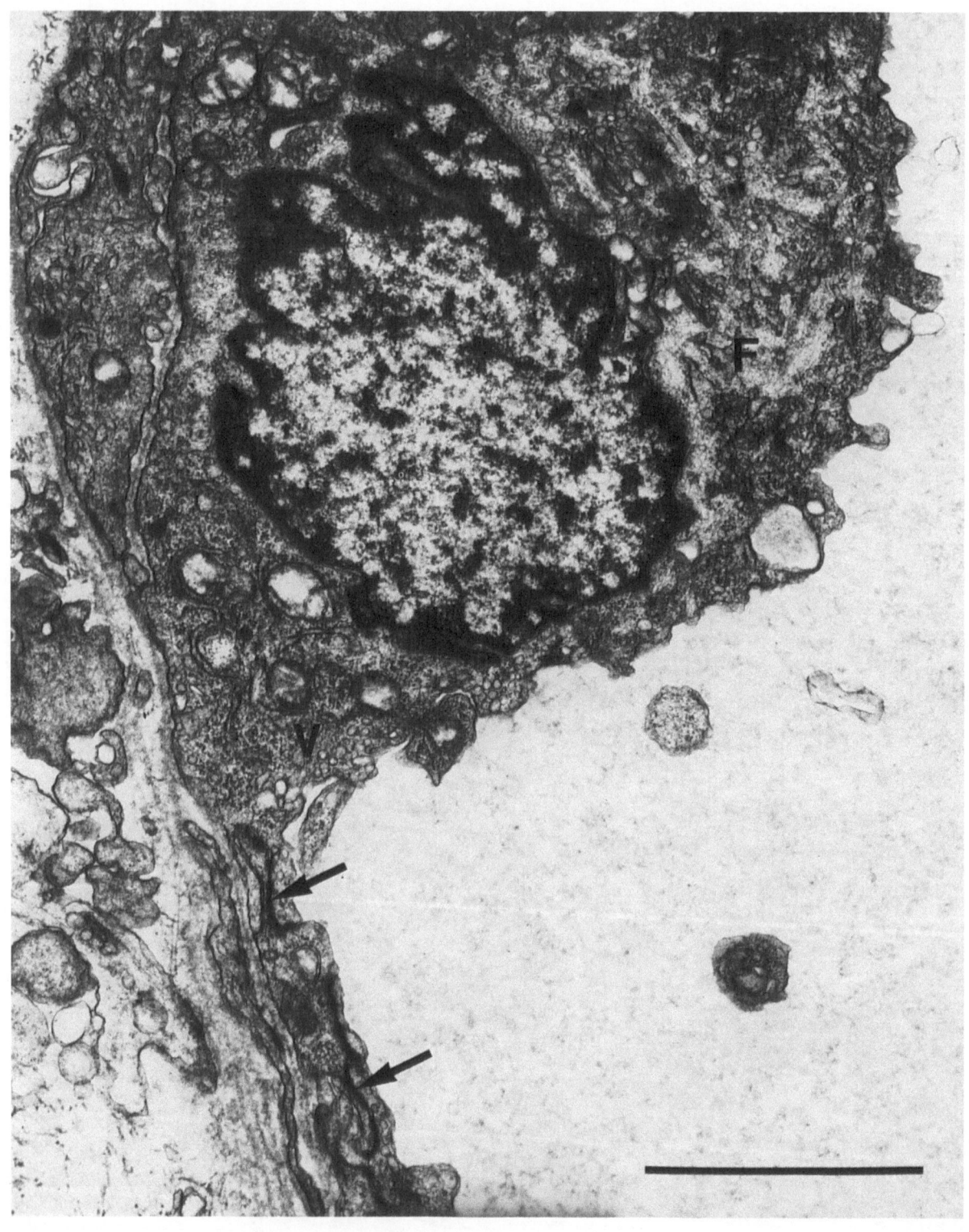

Fig. 17.5. *Haemangioblastoma.* Endothelial cells contain 7-nm filaments (*F*) and abundant pinocytotic vesicles (*V*). Unlike the pericytes, they are linked by elongate desmosomes (*arrows*). An intact, peri-endothelial basement membrane is visible to the *left* of these endothelial cells, with the capillary lumen present on the *right* of the field. (Bar = 2 μm)

18 Germinoma

The ultrastructural appearance of germinomas is very similar to that of testicular seminomas, and they bear no relation to primary pineal tumours despite their typical site in the pineal region. Like seminomas, they are probably of germ cell origin and consist of a population of large neoplastic cells with a second, smaller cell type resembling lymphocytes.

The large tumour cells are usually up to 15 μm across and have abundant, well-defined perikaryal cytoplasm which does not form processes. The nuclei are large and irregular in shape, with pale staining chromatin and prominent nucleoli. The cytoplasm contains only scanty rough endoplasmic reticulum, but there are usually abundant polyribosomes, prominent, large mitochondria and well-developed Golgi bodies. In addition, many cells contain lipid vacuoles and pools of glycogen granules. The latter are often lost during processing, leaving irregular cytoplasmic spaces. As in testicular seminomas, there may also be annulate lamellae in some of the large tumour cells. These structures, which resemble paracrystalline stacks of endoplasmic reticulum, are associated with increased rates of metabolic activity and have been found in a variety of normal and neoplastic cell types. The large tumour cells lack either basement membrane or junctional attachments and are usually separated by abundant extracellular space. This contains mainly collagen and irregular fibroblastic cells, but astrocytic processes filled with 6- to 9-nm glial filaments may also be present towards the edge of the tumour.

The smaller cells present in these tumours are usually less than 6 μm across and have an ultrastructural appearance very similar to small lymphocytes. Their nuclei are round or deeply clefted, with prominent clumping of nuclear chromatin. There is typically only a scanty rim of perinuclear cytoplasm, which is electron dense and largely filled by polyribosomes. These lymphocytic cells do not form junctional attachments and are typically arranged in small, separate clusters. They may also be closely apposed to the larger tumour cells, and in some instances are flattened around the outer surface of these cells or deeply invaginate their cytoplasm. This arrangement has led to the suggestion that the lymphocytic cells are not themselves neoplastic, but represent part of a cell-mediated immune response to the large tumour cells. Large macrophages filled with membrane-bound phagocytic vacuoles have been observed in some cases, and may also be involved in such an immune process.

Further Reading

Cravioto H, Dart D (1973) The ultrastructure of "pinealomas" (seminoma-like tumour of the pineal region). J Neuropathol Exp Neurol 32: 552–565

Ramsey HJ (1965) Ultrastructure of pineal tumour. Cancer 18: 1014–1025

Tabuchi K, Yamada O, Nishimoto A (1973) The ultrastructure of pinealomas. Acta Neuropathol 24: 117–127

Wischnitzer S (1970) The annulate lamellus. Int Rev Cytol 27: 65–100

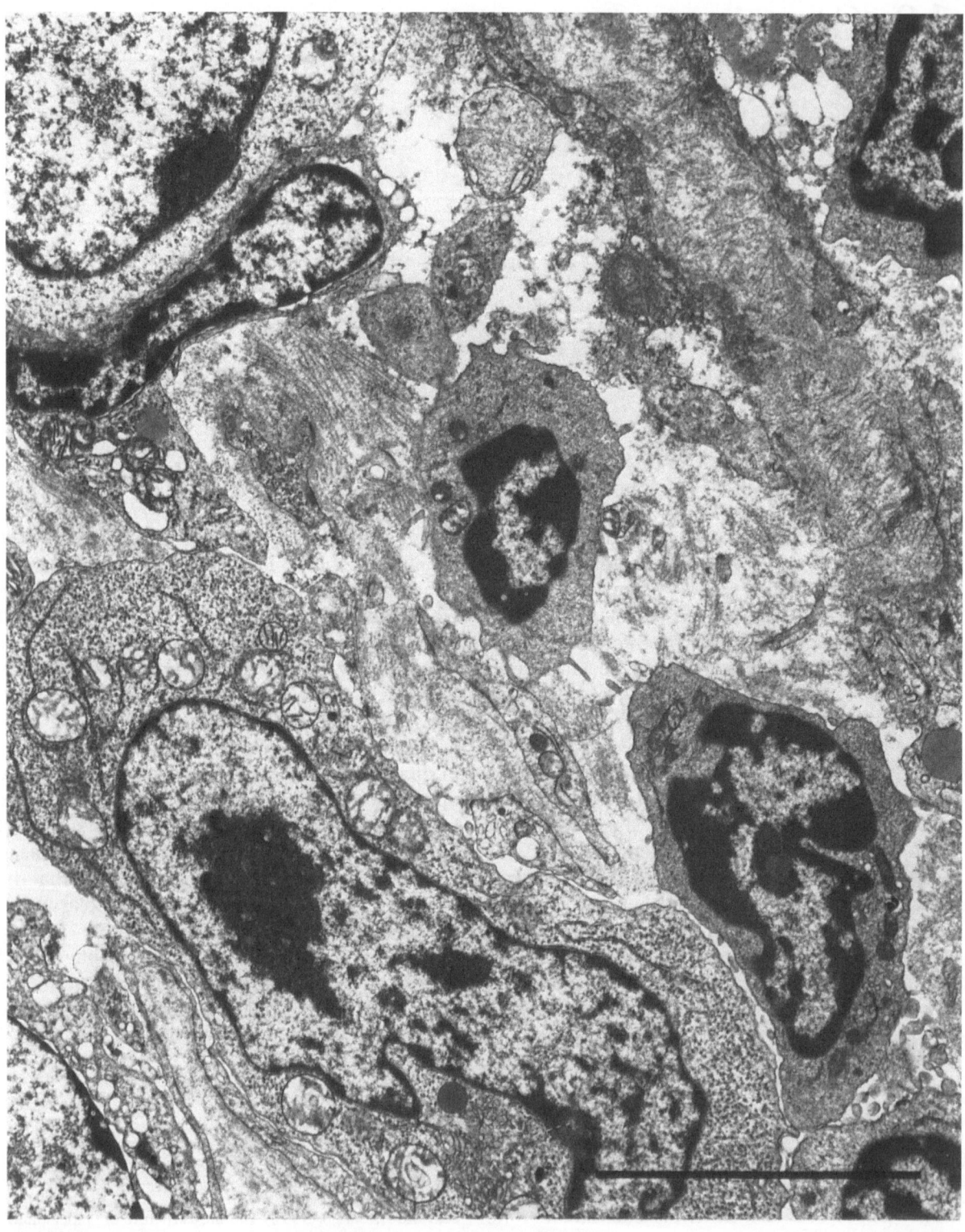

Fig. 18.1. *Germinoma*. The ultrastructural features are very similar to those of testicular seminomas. The large tumour cells, like that seen at the *bottom* of this figure, have irregular nuclei, prominent nucleoli and abundant perinuclear cytoplasm. The smaller, lymphocytic cells may be closely juxtaposed to the large cells, as in the *top left corner*. The abundant extracellular space contains collagen and thin fibroblastic processes. (Bar = 5 μm)

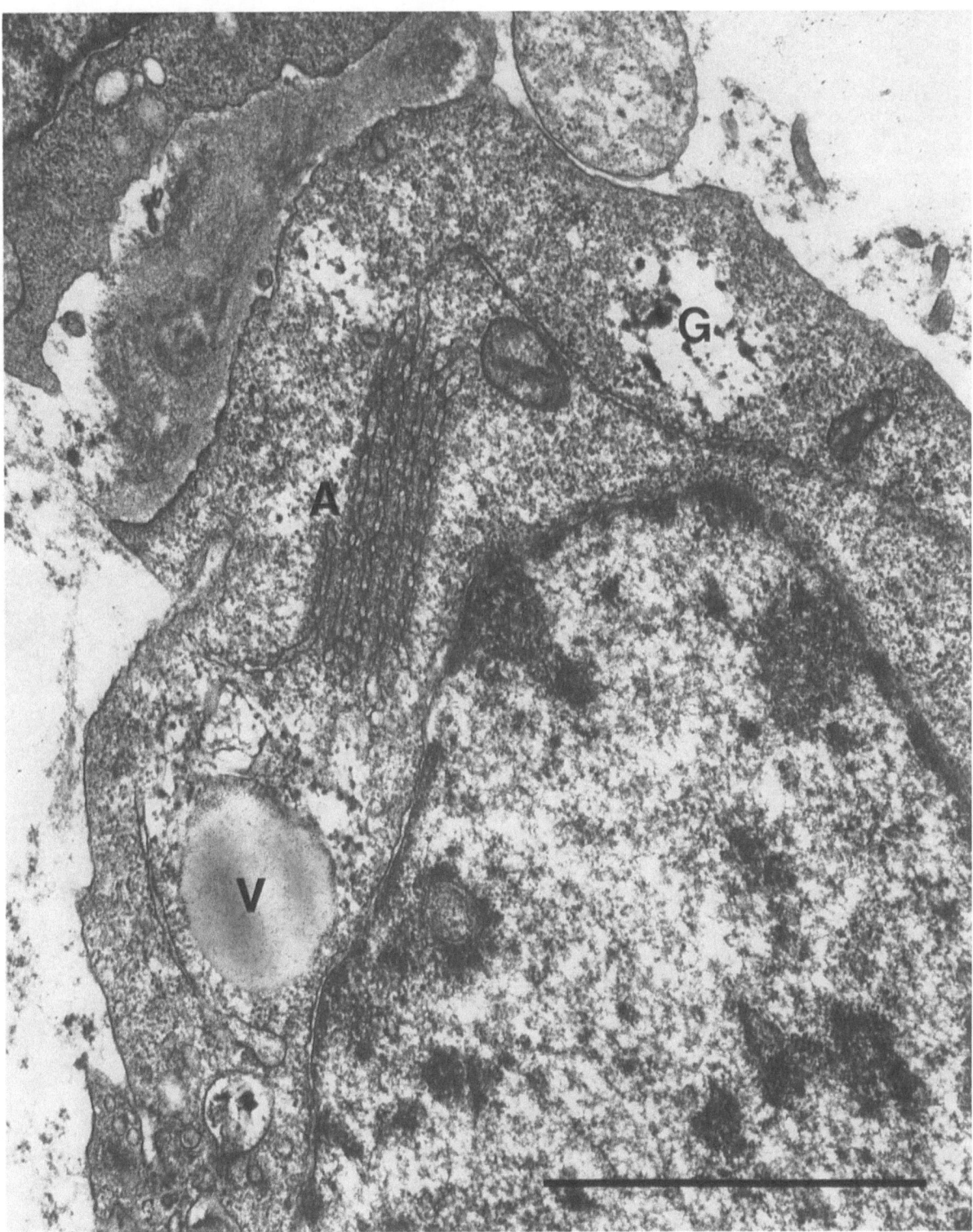

Fig. 18.2. *Germinoma.* The large tumour cells have cytoplasm filled by abundant polyribosomes and may occasionally contain annulate lamellae (*A*). These structures resemble paracrystalline stacks of endoplasmic reticulum and are associated with increased rates of cell metabolism, especially in germ cells. Other cytoplasmic structures which may be present include lipid vacuoles (*V*) and pools of glycogen granules. The latter are often depleted during processing, leaving irregular cytoplasmic spaces like the one seen in this cell (*G*). (Bar = 2 μm)

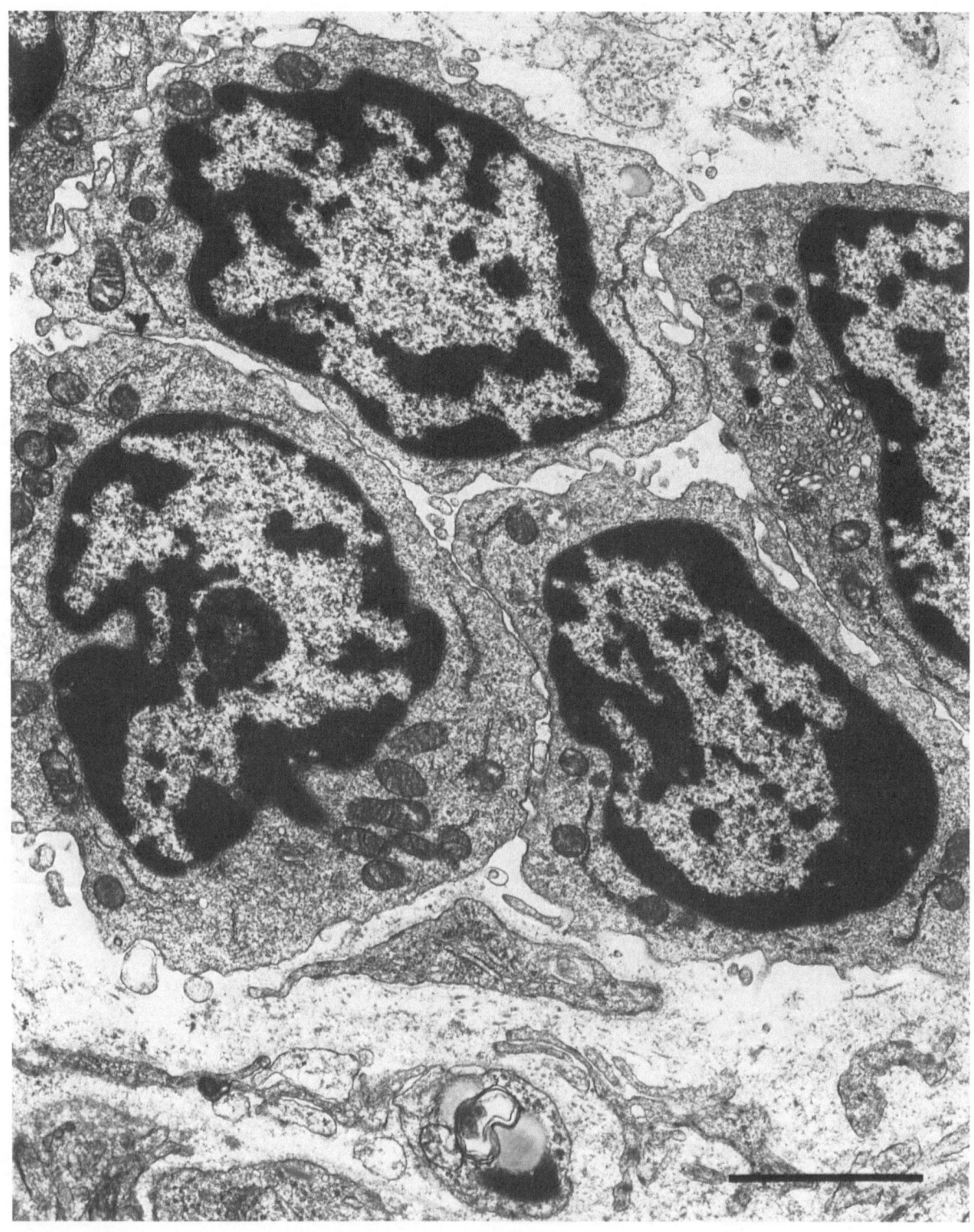

Fig. 18.3. *Germinoma.* The small cells present in these tumours are ultrastructurally identical to small lymphocytes and are often arranged in small, separate clusters like the one shown here. They have rounded or clefted nuclei and only a thin rim of electron-dense cytoplasm, largely filled by polyribosomes. (Bar = 2 μm)

19 Craniopharyngioma

Craniopharyngiomas are largely composed of epithelioid cell masses with an ultrastructural appearance very similar to the stratum spinosum of normal skin. The tumour cells have irregular, ovoid nuclei containing one or more prominent nucleoli, and are joined by numerous, well-defined desmosomes. The relatively scanty perinuclear cytoplasm generally contains rather sparse organelles but there are prominent masses of 5-nm tonofilaments. These are sometimes grouped into separate, electron-dense bundles, which are visible as "keratohyaline granules" on light microscopy.

Towards the periphery of each epithelioid mass, the cells have a more polygonal shape and the relatively narrow intercellular spaces are bridged by numerous, short, microvillous processes. An intact basement membrane separates the outer basaloid layer of cells from the extra-epithelioid cystic spaces. In more central areas, the cells have a stellate shape and are widely separated by abundant extracellular space. The cells in these areas are connected by long, tenuous processes, which are joined to each other at their distal ends by desmosomes. The pockets of extracellular space enclosed by these processes are lined by an irregular, broad zone of amorphous, basement membrane-like material, which is closely applied to the cell membranes.

The areas outside the epithelioid cell masses take the form of large cystic spaces, lined by the basaloid layer of tumour cells and their basement membrane. These spaces normally contain mesenchymal elements, including collagen and blood vessels. Towards the periphery of the tumour, however, there may also be abundant astrocytic cells and processes containing 6- to 9-nm glial filaments and Rosenthal bodies (see Chap. 1). Within the epithelioid cell masses, there are other, usually much smaller, cystic spaces. These are lined by flattened tumour cells which contain abundant 5-nm tonofilaments and have microvilli on their luminal surfaces. The central cavities contain dense masses of amorphous and fine fibrillary material, which represent the ultrastructural equivalent of keratin. Cellular debris, including fragmented desmosomes, may also be present within these intra-epithelioid cysts and they appear to be formed following the degeneration of one or more central tumour cells. In some of these tumours there may also be numerous electron-dense, amorphous masses of calcified material, both between tumour cells and within the larger intra-epithelioid cysts.

Further Reading

Ghatak NR, Hirano A, Zimmerman HM (1971) Ultrastructure of a craniopharyngioma. Cancer 27: 1465–1475

Landolt AM (1975) Ultrastructure of human sella tumours. Correlations of clinical findings and morphology. 7: Craniopharyngiomas. Acta Neuropathol [Suppl] 22: 104–119

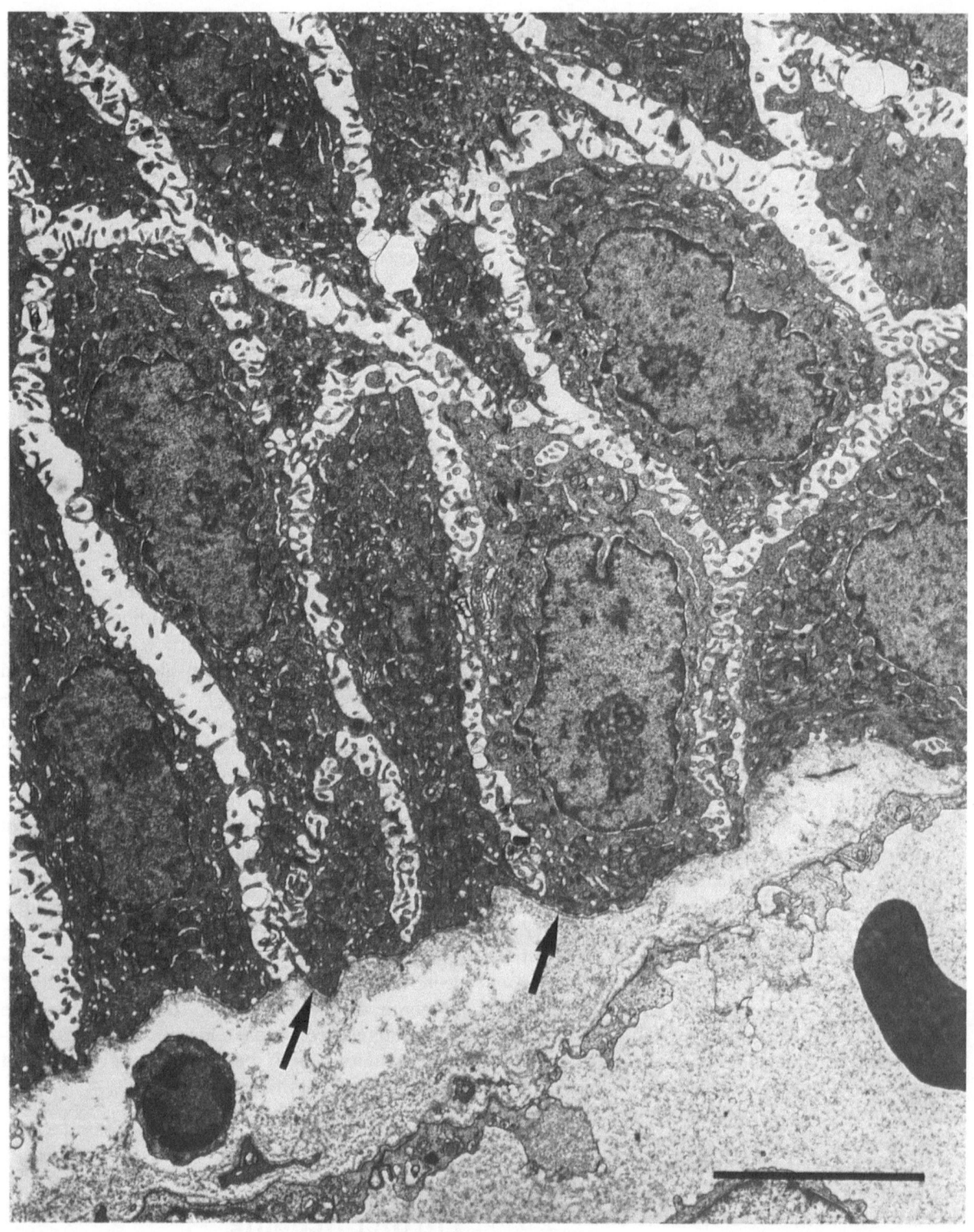

Fig. 19.1. *Craniopharyngioma.* Towards the edges of the epithelioid cell masses, the tumour cells are polygonal in shape, like those seen here. The narrow intercellular spaces are bridged by numerous, short microvillous processes. An intact, outer basement membrane (*arrows*) separates the basaloid, outermost cell layer from large cystic areas. These contain collagen and blood vessels, such as the one occupying the *lower right corner* of this figure. (Bar = 5 μm)

124

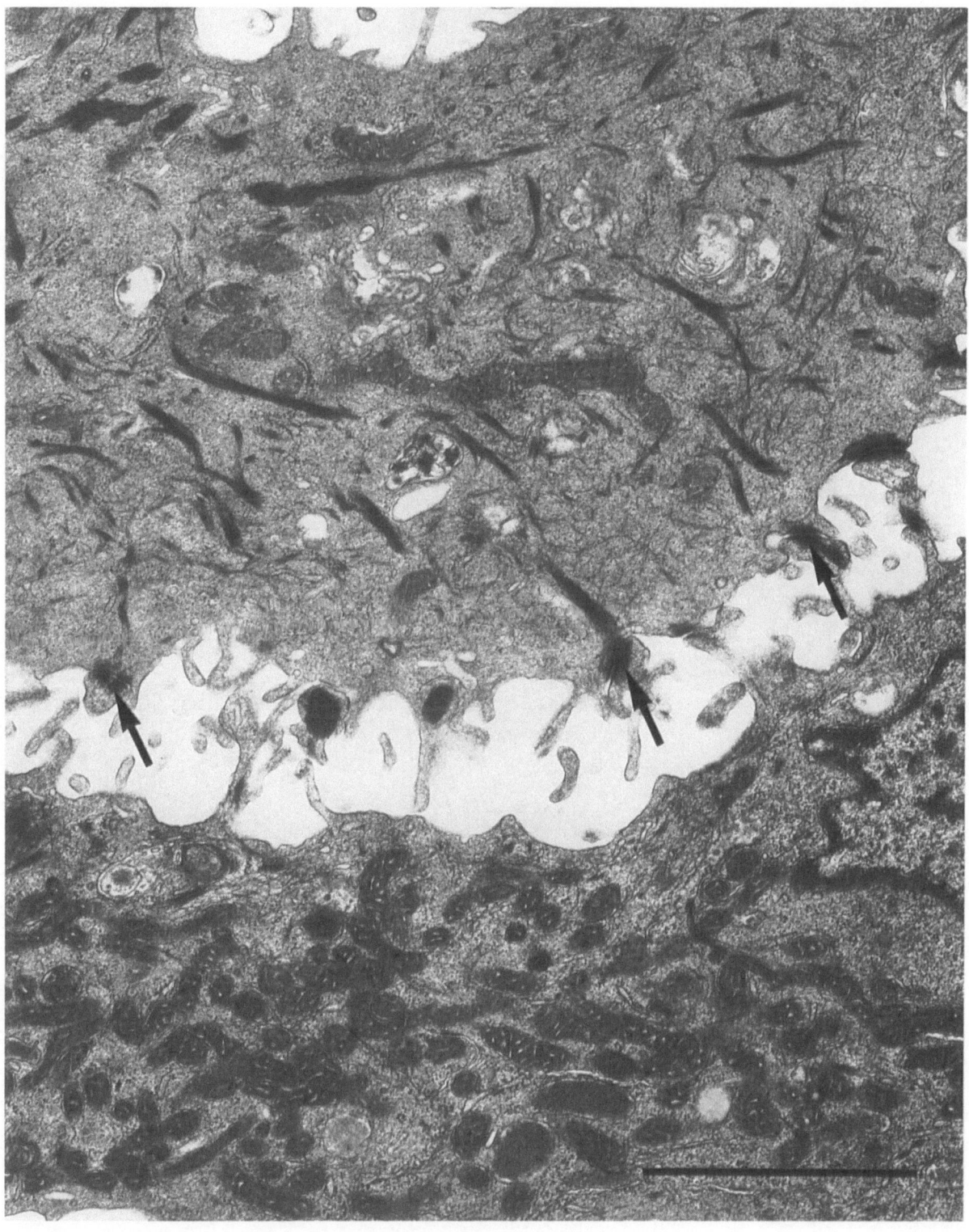

Fig. 19.2. *Craniopharyngioma.* Adjacent cells are joined by numerous, well-defined desmosomes (*arrows*). The cell cytoplasm usually contains abundant 5-nm tonofilaments, which may be grouped into separate, electron-dense bundles, as in the uppermost of the two cells here. These bundles are visible as keratohyaline granules on light microscopy. (Bar = 2 μm)

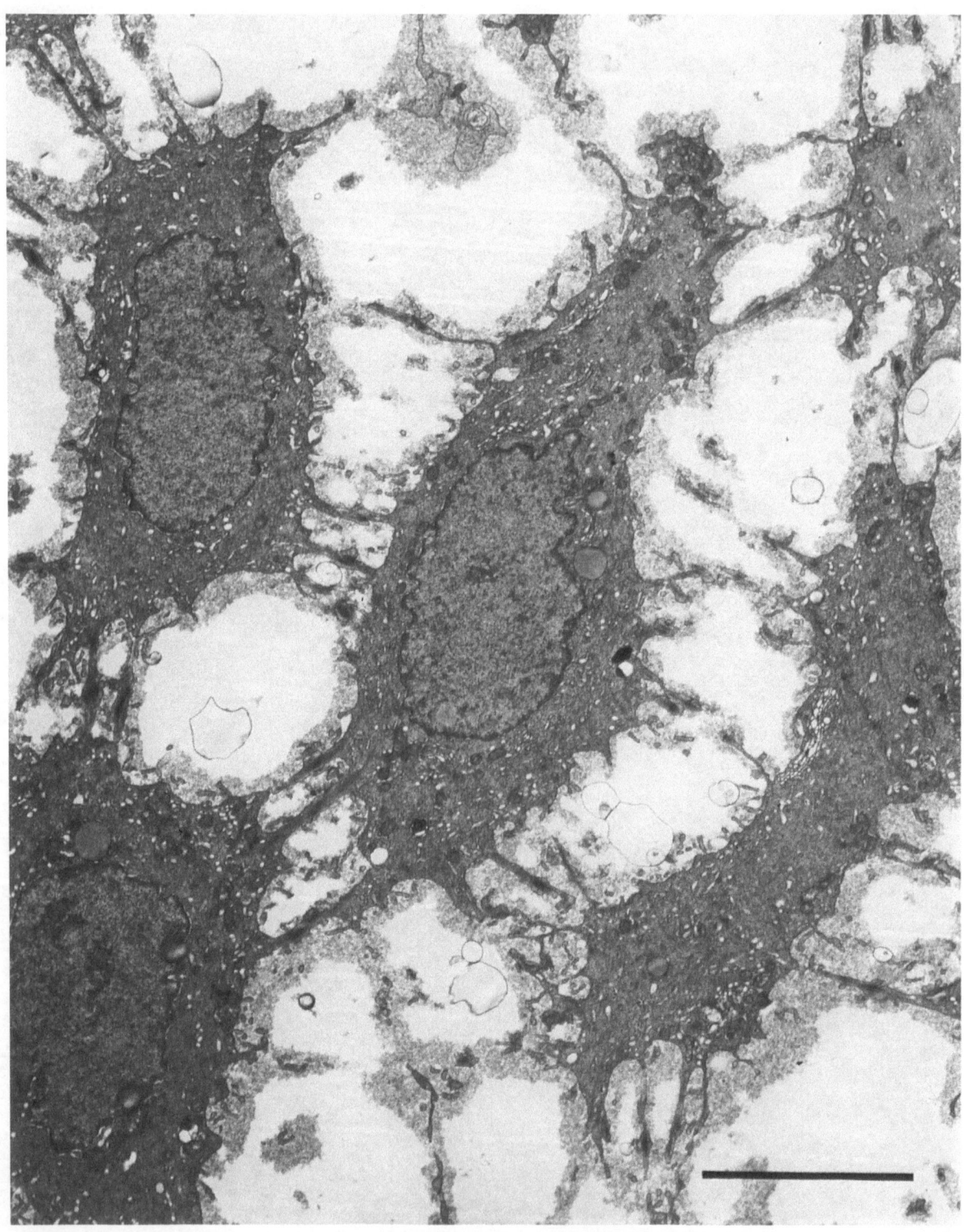

Fig. 19.3. *Craniopharyngioma*. Towards the centre of each epithelioid cell mass, the tumour cell bodies are more widely spaced and stellate in shape, like those illustrated here. They are connected by tenuous cell processes which enclose separate loculi of extracellular space. These enclosed areas are lined by irregular but broad zones of amorphous, basement membrane-like material, which is a prominent feature in this field. (Bar = 5 μm)

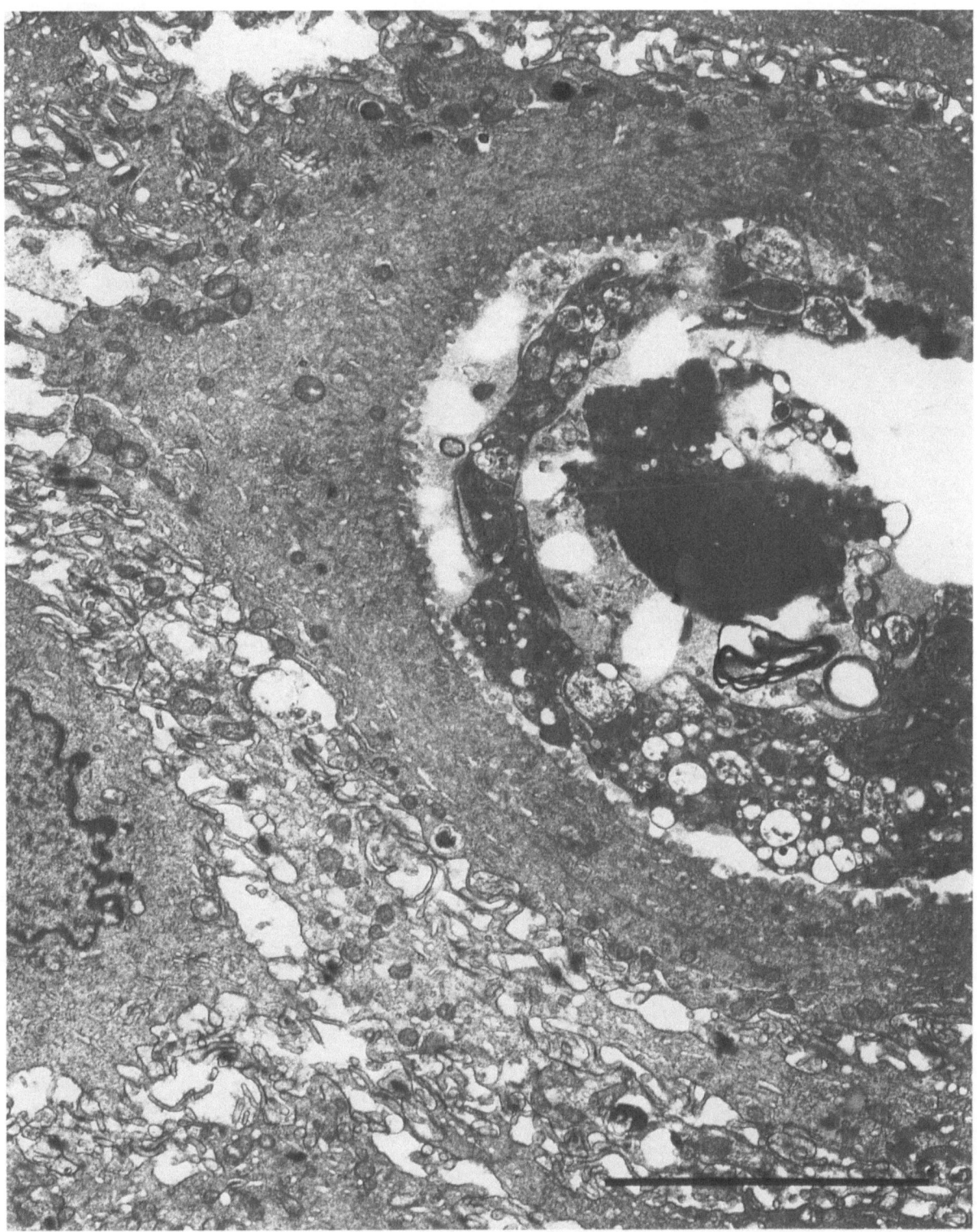

Fig. 19.4. *Craniopharyngioma.* Intra-epithelial cysts, like the one on the *right*, are enclosed by flattened cells with luminal microvilli and abundant 5-nm tonofilaments in their cytoplasm. As in the example shown here, these cysts usually contain a variety of cell debris, together with the osmiophilic fibrillary material which represents keratin. (Bar = 5 μm)

20 Chordoma

Chordomas are rare tumours which are thought to be derived from embryonic notochord remnants persisting within the spinal column, and they typically arise either at the sacral end of the column or in the region of the foramen magnum. The tumour cells are arranged in irregular cords or clumps, often widely separated by large extracellular spaces. The mucinous material present in these spaces consists ultrastructurally of dense, granular or fibrillary material, which is often condensed around the tumour cell surfaces. Distinct basement membranes, however, are an inconstant feature and are patchy or entirely absent in many cases. Intercellular junctions are generally rather infrequent, but occasional zonulae occludens or desmosomes may be present where adjacent cells are closely packed together. In many areas, the tumour cells show a marked tendency to form numerous short and irregular cytoplasmic processes, or pseudopodia. These may project from free cell surfaces and resemble blunt microvilli, but they more typically form a complex, interdigitating meshwork between closely apposed tumour cell bodies.

The tumour cells generally have abundant cytoplasm and lobulated or deeply indented nuclei with prominent nucleoli. The smallest cells present, often referred to as stellate cells, are irregular in shape and lack cytoplasmic vacuoles. The larger "physaliphorous" cells have cell bodies distended by numerous giant intracytoplasmic vacuoles, which are often enclosed by only a thin rim of flattened cytoplasm. Between these two extremes there is a spectrum of cell types showing intermediate degrees of vacuolation, and the overall appearances are thought to represent a single population of tumour cells undergoing progressive cytoplasmic vacuolation. The vacuoles may contain granular or fibrillary material similar to that in the extracellular space, but often appear entirely empty. Other cytoplasmic organelles include prominent Golgi bodies, bundles of 7- to 10-nm intermediate filaments and abundant pinocytotic vesicles. In addition, many cells contain glycogen granules, either scattered throughout the cytoplasm or enclosed within small vacuoles. There are also numerous short cisternae of rough endoplasmic reticulum, which are often dilated and occasionally contain elongate, paracrystalline inclusions. The most characteristic ultrastructural feature of chordomas, however, is the presence of cytoplasmic organelle complexes. These are formed from mitochondria and cisternae of rough endoplasmic reticulum, which alternate with each other in a structurally ordered fashion and are separated by a constant, narrow gap of approximately 50 nm. Such complexes are not an entirely specific feature, since similar structures have been produced experimentally in animals, but they may be useful in distinguishing chordomas from other mucinous tumours, such as secondary adenocarcinomas.

Further Reading

Dolman CL (1984) Ultrastructure of brain tumours and biopsies. Praeger, New York, pp 85–105

Erlandson RA, Tandler B, Lieberman PM, Higinbotham NO (1968) Ultrastructure of human chordoma. Cancer Res 28: 2115–2125

Ho K-L (1985) Eccordosis physaliphora and chordoma: a comparative ultrastructural study. Clin Neuropathol 4: 77–86

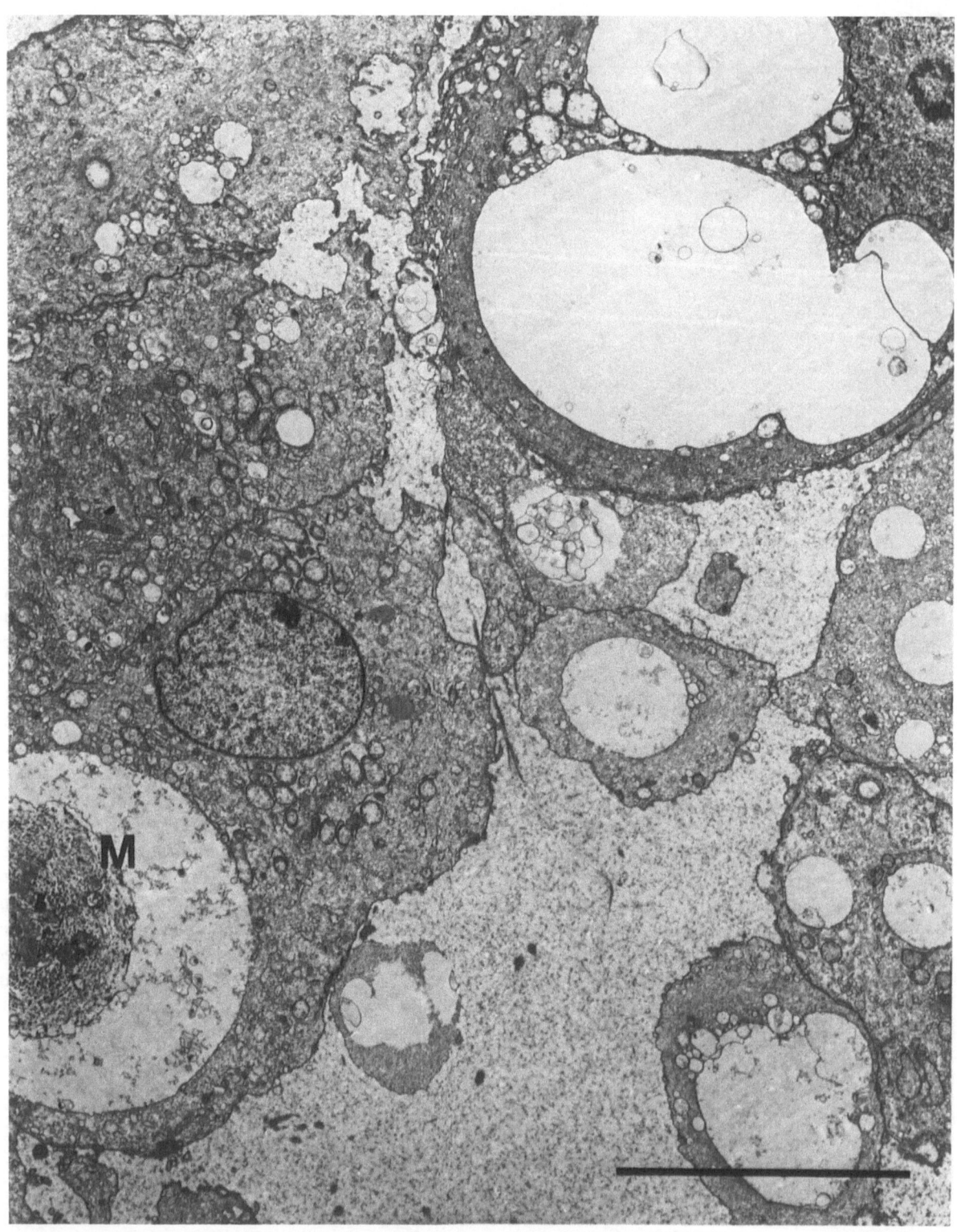

Fig. 20.1. *Chordoma.* The tumour cells are arranged in irregular clumps separated by abundant extracellular space. Larger, "physaliphorous" cells, like that seen in the *upper right corner*, have cell bodies distended by numerous giant vacuoles, often enclosed by only a thin rim of cytoplasm. Other tumour cells present (sometimes called intermediate cells) show a widely varying spectrum of less severe vacuolar change. The vacuoles often appear empty, but sometimes contain granular or fibrillary material (*M*) similar to that present in the extracellular space. (Bar = 10 μm)

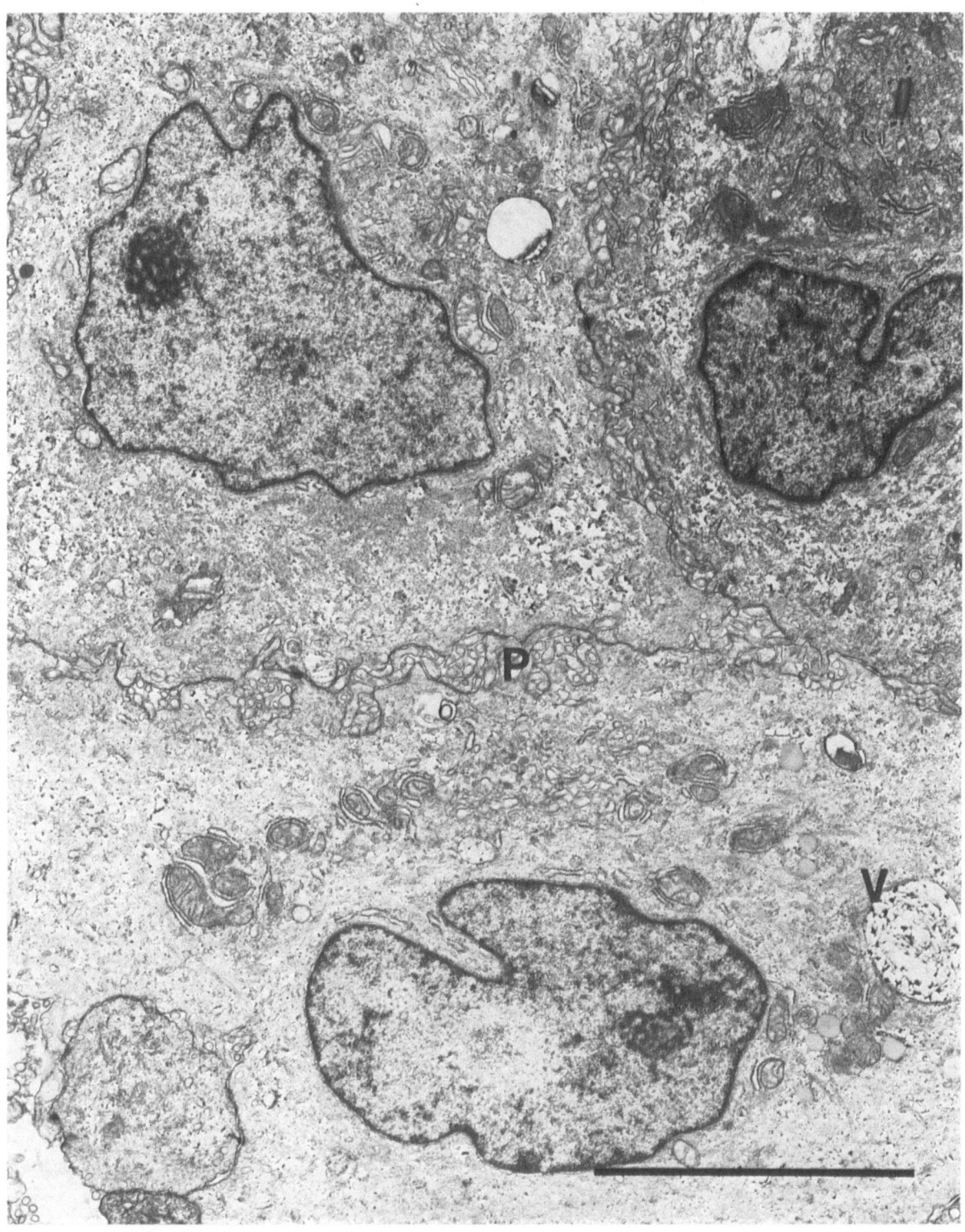

Fig. 20.2. *Chordoma.* Nuclei are often deeply indented and usually contain a prominent nucleolus. Smaller, or "stellate" tumour cells, like those in this field, lack large cytoplasmic vacuoles but are otherwise similar to the "physaliphorous" cells. Electron-dense glycogen granules may lie free within the cytoplasm, as in the uppermost cells here, or within small vacuoles (*V*). Adjacent cells are frequently attached to each other by a complex meshwork of short cytoplasmic processes, or pseudopodia (*P*). (Bar = 5 μm)

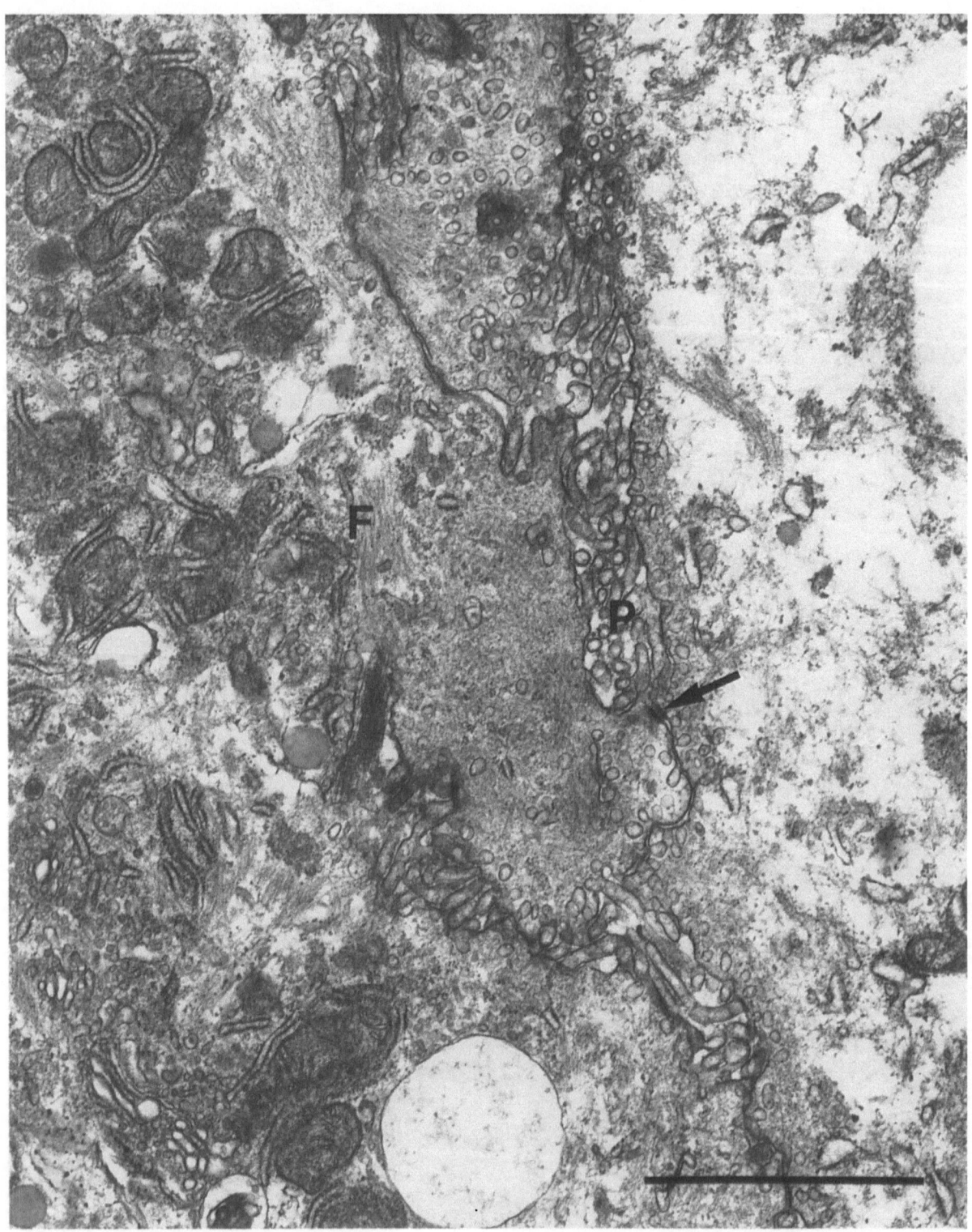

Fig. 20.3. *Chordoma.* The cytoplasmic organelle complexes typical of this tumour are seen in the *upper left* of this field. They consist of mitochondria and cisternae of rough endoplasmic reticulum alternating in a structurally ordered fashion. The tumour cell cytoplasm also contains prominent bundles of 7- to 10-nm intermediate filaments (*F*) and often forms a peripheral meshwork of short cytoplasmic processes, or pseudopodia (*P*). Closely apposed cells may be joined by occasional zonulae adherentes or desmosomes (*arrow*) in some areas. (Bar = 2 μm)

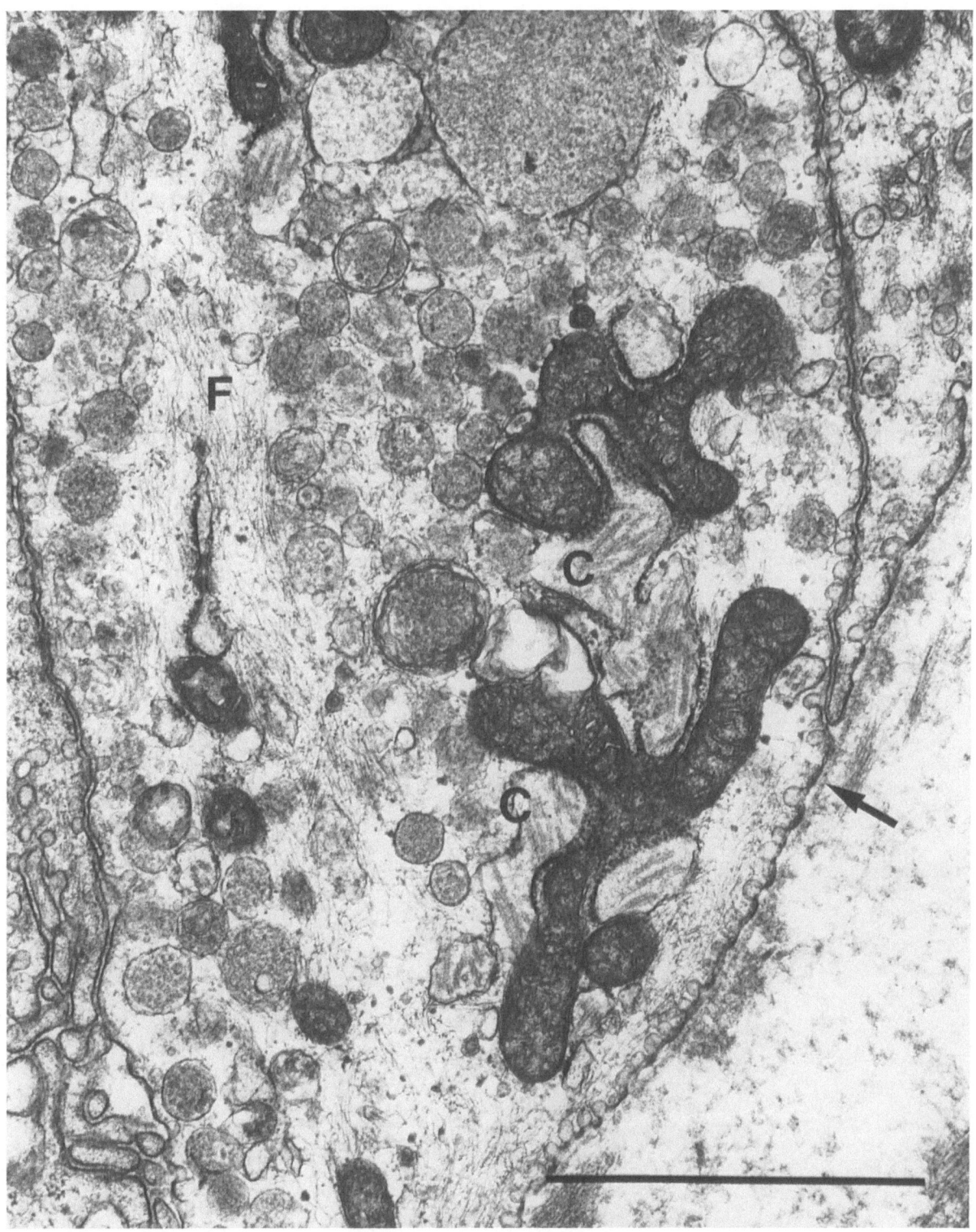

Fig. 20.4. *Chordoma.* Cisternae of rough endoplasmic reticulum are often dilated, like those in the organelle complexes seen here, and occasionally contain elongate, paracrystalline structures (*C*). Pinocytotic vesicles are usually abundant, as around the margins of these cells, but basement membrane (*arrow*) is patchy and often entirely absent. 7- to 10-nm intermediate filaments are clearly visible in the cytoplasm of this cell (*F*). The extracellular mucinous substance, visible in the *lower right corner*, has a granular or finely fibrillar appearance at ultrastructural level. (Bar = 2 μm)

21 Pituitary Adenoma

All these tumours have a basically similar appearance at electron microscopic level, and although the various secretory subtypes may show individual characteristic features, they cannot be reliably distinguished from each other on purely ultrastructural grounds.

The tumour cells are typically polygonal and closely packed together in sheets. There are no peripheral processes and the cells do not usually form junctional attachments. The nuclei are often deeply indented and may contain prominent nucleoli. The abundant cytoplasm has a very varied organelle population, but most cells contain membrane-bound neurosecretory granules, often arranged in rows just under the cell membranes. The granules are very variable in size, and although their mean diameter is probably dependent on the secretory type of the tumour, this relationship is not consistent or well defined. Actively secreting cells typically contain abundant rough endoplasmic reticulum and Golgi apparatus but relatively few secretory granules, whereas inactive or storage-type cells tend to show the reverse picture, with abundant granules. Concentric arrays of endoplasmic reticulum, or "Nebenkern", may be a prominent feature in some tumours. Extracellular collagen is sparse and capillary vessels usually have thin, fenestrated endothelial walls.

Amyloid is most common in growth hormone or prolactin-secreting tumours and consists ultrastructurally of irregular masses of 7- to 10-nm filamentous material. It may occur within tumour cell cytoplasm or in the perivascular spaces. In some instances it forms large, paracrystalline bodies, with radiating bundles of filaments enclosed by flattened, degenerate-looking cells.

Tumours secreting growth hormone show much greater nuclear and cellular pleomorphism than other types and usually have very abundant neurosecretory granules of widely varying size. Prolactin-secreting tumours have relatively few, intermediate sized granules, with a maximum diameter of about 200 nm. They may show misplaced exocytosis, in which extruded granules are trapped between closely apposed cell bodies. A dual population of light and dark cell types has been described in tumours secreting both prolactin and growth hormone together. Tumours secreting ACTH typically have abundant, large granules, often more than 400 nm across. In cells undergoing Crooke's hyaline degeneration, the swollen cytoplasm is filled by abundant, tangled 7-nm filaments, together with lysosomal vacuoles and amorphous material resembling lipofuscin. Granules and other cytoplasmic organelles are displaced or depleted in these cells, and there may be disintegration of the plasma membrane. This change is thought to represent either overproduction or failed degradation of filaments normally present in the cells, but the relationship of this material to amyloid is uncertain. In nonsecretory tumours, the neurosecretory granules are very sparse and small, with an outer diameter usually less than 100 nm. Other organelles also tend to be very scanty, but in some cases the cells may show oncocytic change, in which the cytoplasm is entirely filled by abundant mitochondria.

Further Reading

DeCicco A, Dekker A, Yunis EJ (1972) Fine structure of Crooke's hyaline change in the human pituitary gland. Arch Pathol 94: 65–70

Doniach I (1972) Cytology of pituitary adenomas. J R Coll Physicians 6: 299–308

Esiri MM, Adams CBT, Burke C, Underdown R (1983) Pituitary adenomas: immunohistology and ultrastructural analysis of 118 tumours. Acta Neuropathol 62: 1–14

Landolt AM (1975) Ultrastructure of human sella tumours. Correlations of clinical findings and morphology. Acta Neurochir [Suppl] 22: 1–167

Schober R, Nelson D (1975) Fine structure and origin of amyloid deposits in pituitary adenoma. Arch Pathol 99: 403–410

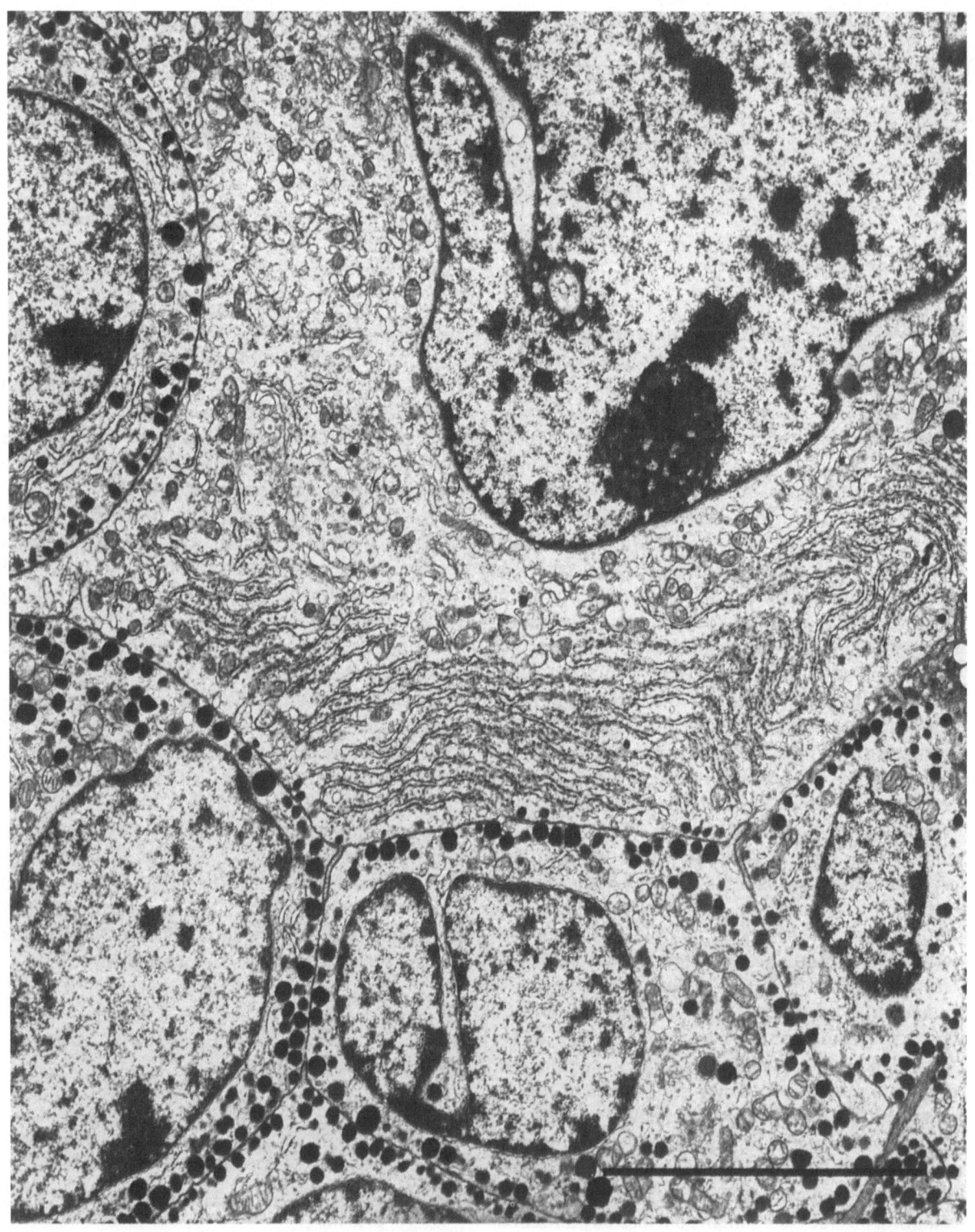

Fig. 21.1. *Pituitary adenoma.* The tumour cells are typically polygonal and closely packed in sheets, like the ones in this ACTH-secreting tumour. The nuclei may show deep clefts and the cytoplasm of most cells contains membrane-bound neurosecretory granules. These are often arranged in rows just beneath the plasma membranes, as in the cells illustrated here. Actively secreting cells, such as that at the *top* of this figure, contain abundant rough endoplasmic reticulum and Golgi apparatus but relatively scanty neurosecretory granules. (Bar = 5 μm)

136

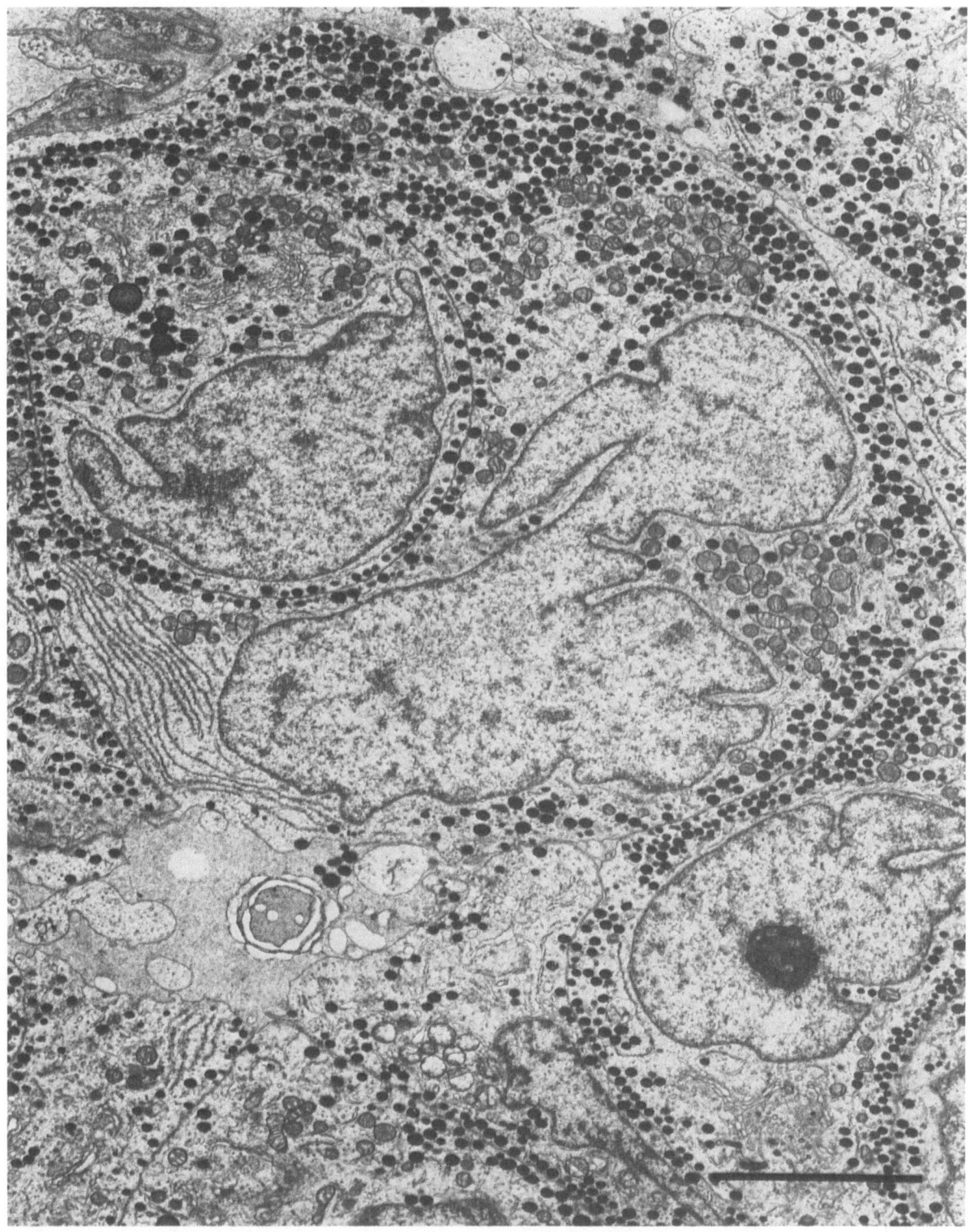

Fig. 21.2. *Pituitary adenoma.* This tumour secreted growth hormone, and shows the marked increase in nuclear and cellular pleomorphism typical of its secretory type. The neurosecretory granules are visible only as black dots at this magnification. They are usually abundant in these tumours, but very variable in size, with diameters between 100 nm and 350 nm. (Bar = 5 μm)

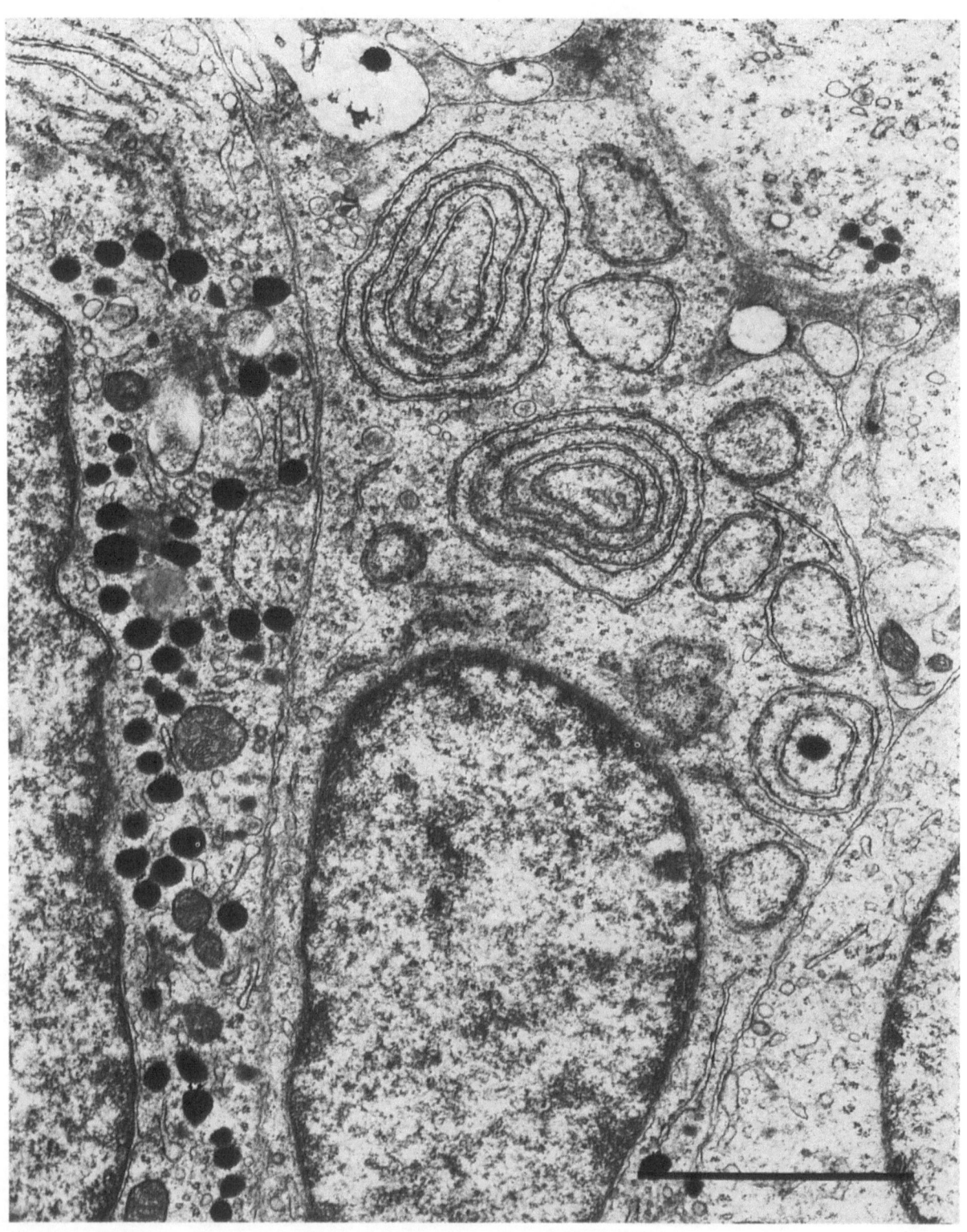

Fig. 21.3. *Pituitary adenoma.* Concentric arrays of endoplasmic reticulum, like those seen here, may be a prominent feature of any secretory type and have been called "Nebenkern". This tumour secreted both growth hormone and prolactin. As in most pituitary adenomas, the plasma membranes of these cells are closely apposed to each other but lack junctional attachments. (Bar = 2 μm)

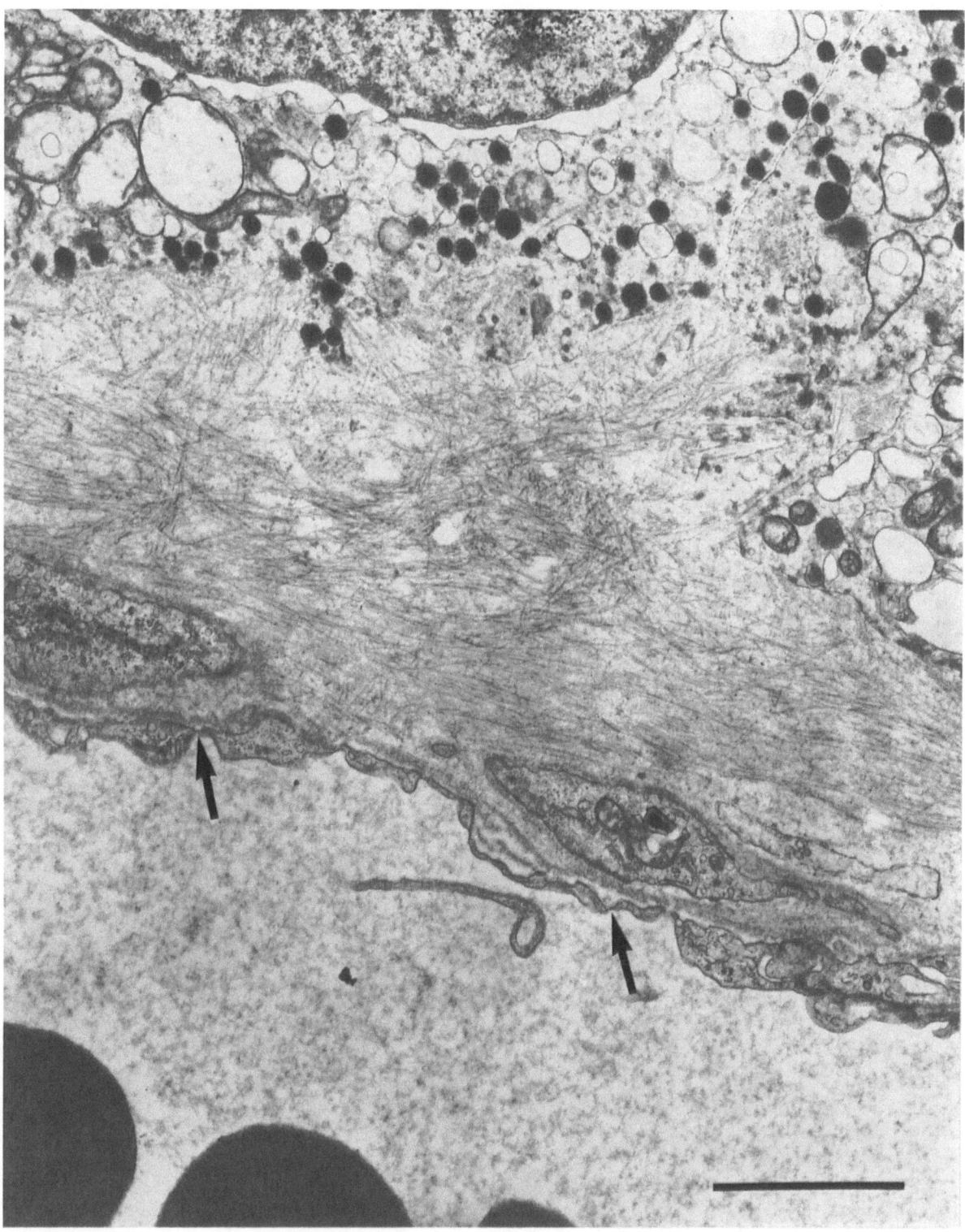

Fig. 21.4. *Pituitary adenoma.* Amyloid is most commonly found in tumours secreting growth hormone or prolactin, and both hormones were present in the tumour illustrated here. It consists ultrastructurally of irregular masses of filamentous material 7- to 10-nm in diameter, and may be intracytoplasmic or lie in the perivascular space, as in the example shown here. The adjacent capillary endothelium is thin and fenestrated (*arrows*) and typical of the vascular endothelium found in most pituitary adenomas. (Bar = 2 μm)

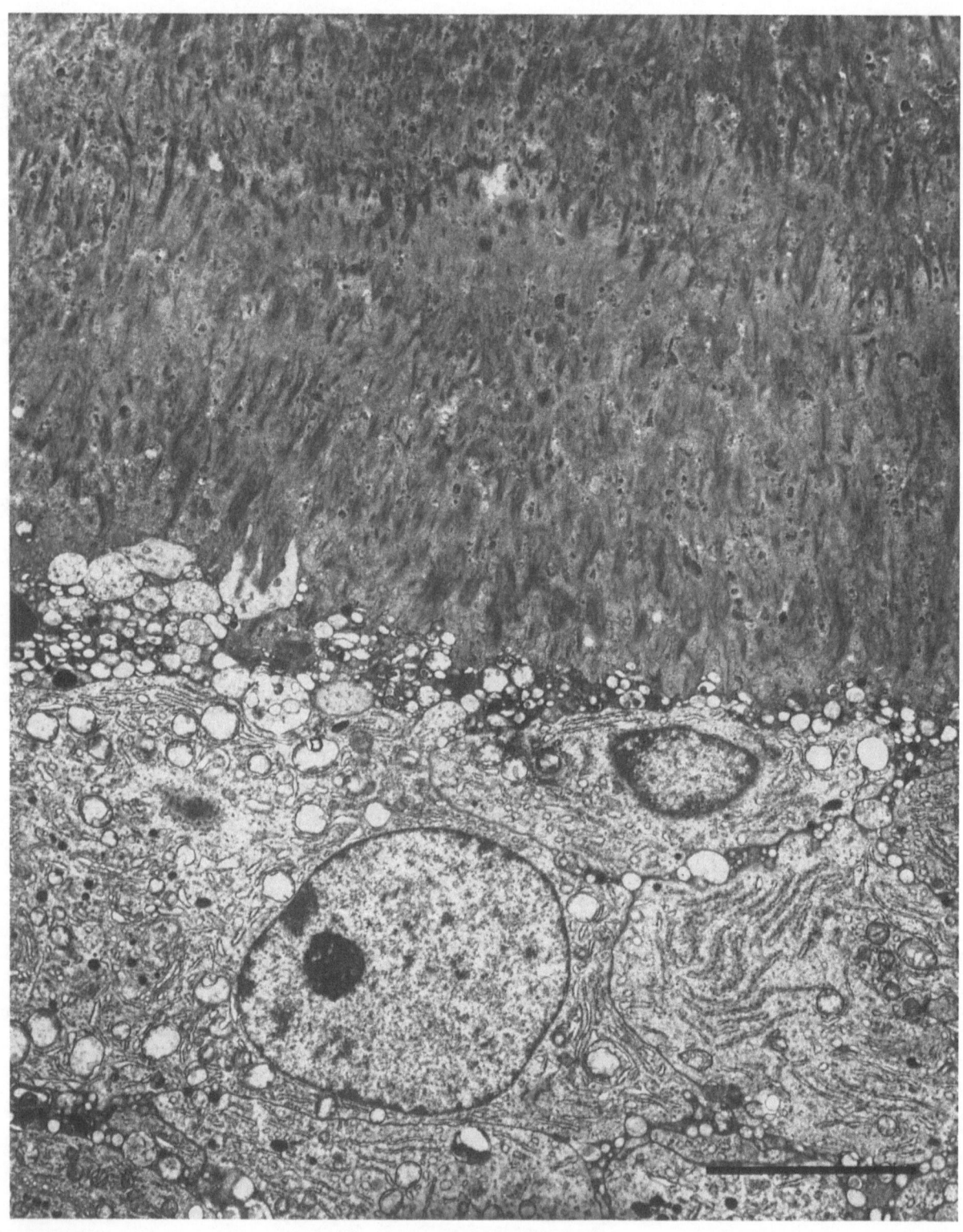

Fig. 21.5. *Pituitary adenoma.* In some instances, the amyloid may form large, paracrystalline bodies, like that occupying the *upper half* of this field. These bodies consist of concentric layers of radiating filament bundles, and are enclosed by a flattened layer of vacuolated, degenerate-looking cells. This tumour secreted prolactin. (Bar = 5 μm)

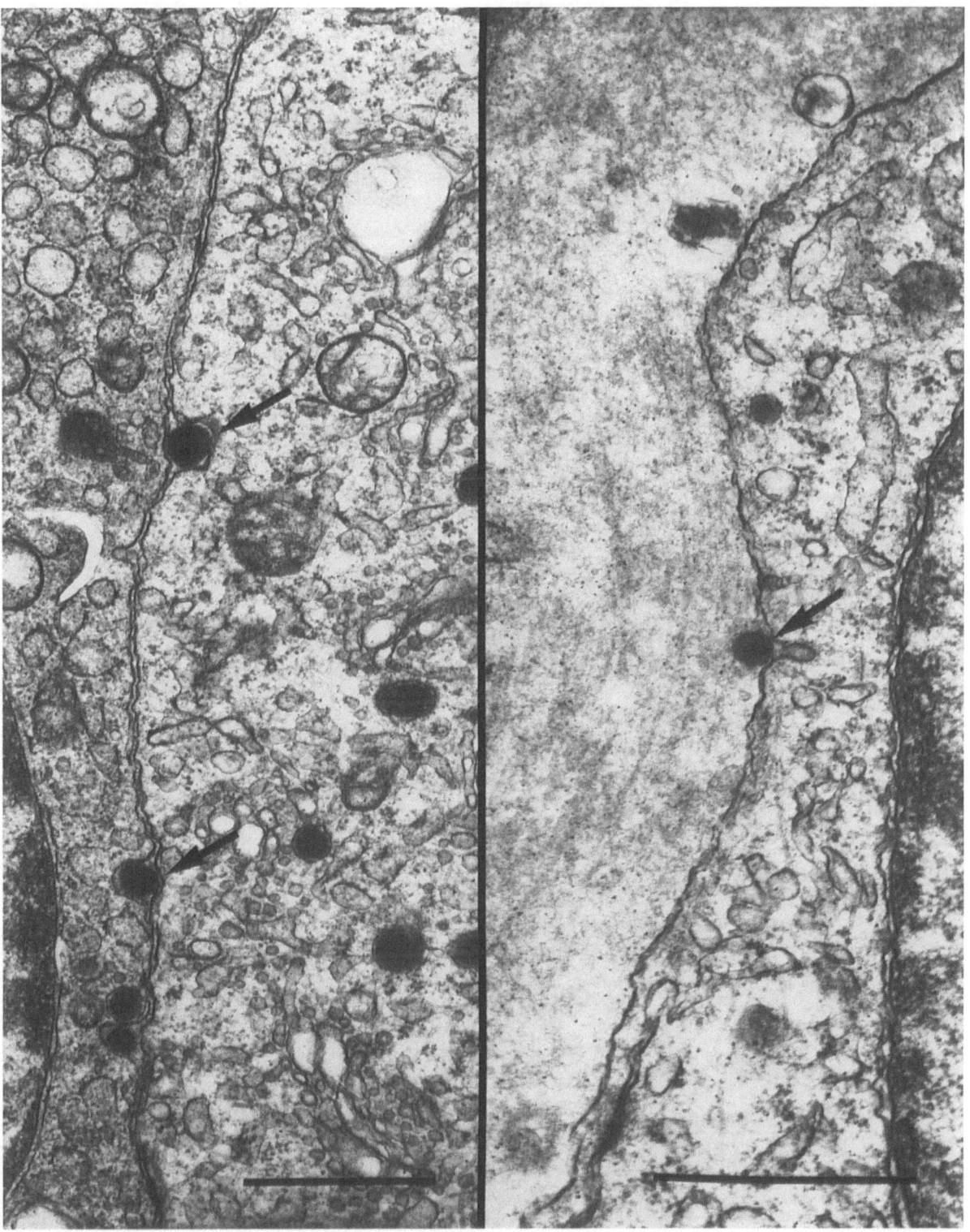

Fig. 21.6. *Pituitary adenoma.* Misplaced exocytosis, shown on the *left*, is a characteristic feature of tumours secreting prolactin. The extruded neurosecretory granules are trapped between closely apposed tumour cells (*arrows*). The outer membrane of the remaining *intra*cytoplasmic granules is clearly visible at this magnification. (Bar = 1 μm). More normal exocytosis is shown on the *right*, with the released granule free in the extracellular space. (Bar = 1 μm)

141

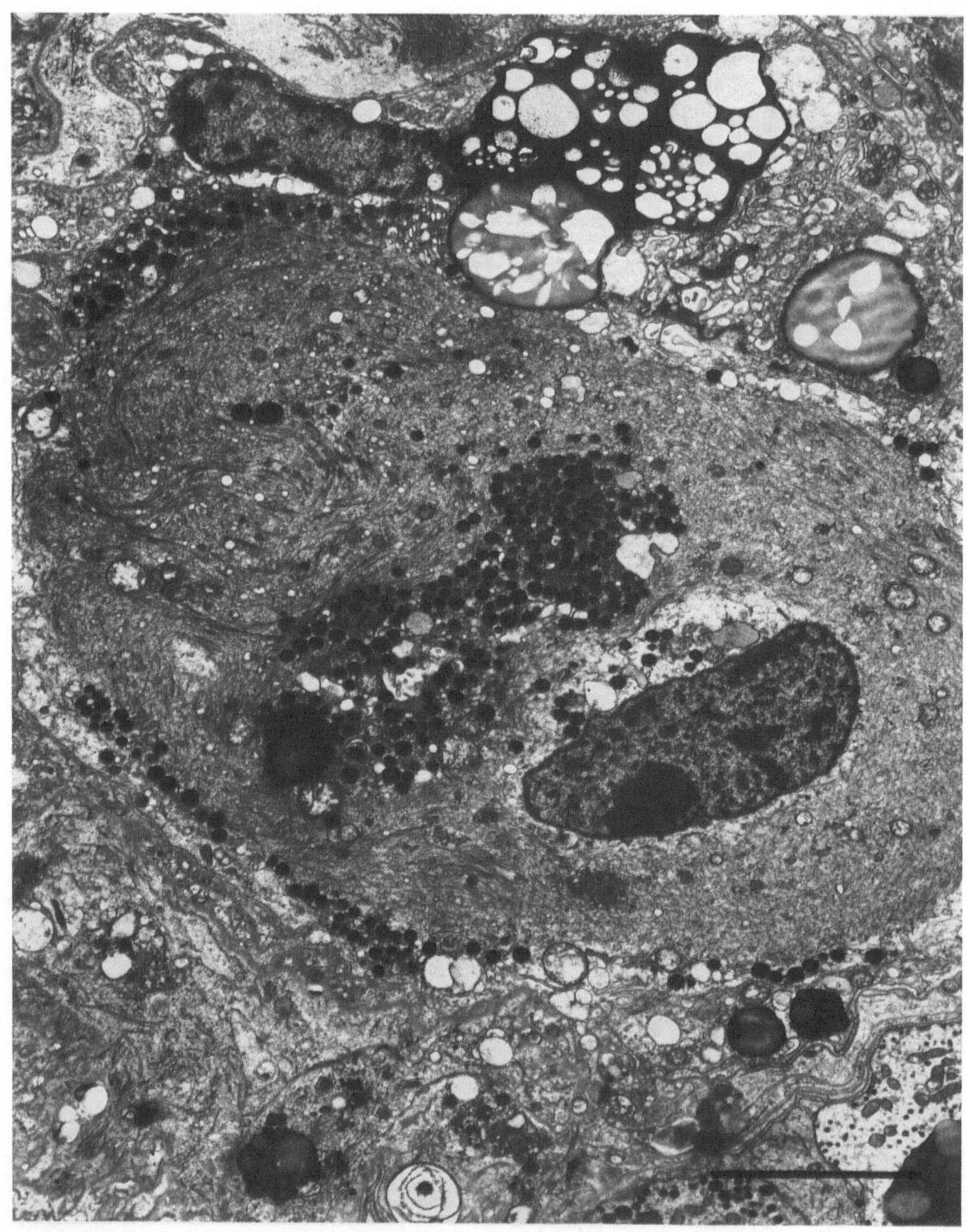

Fig. 21.7. *Pituitary adenoma.* ACTH-secreting tumour. In Crooke's hyaline degeneration, the cytoplasm is distended by abundant 7-nm diameter filamentous material. As in the example shown here, secretory granules are often depleted and displaced to the perinuclear region. Lysosomal vacuoles and osmiophilic material resembling lipofuscin may also be present, like that seen in the degenerate cell at the *very top* of this figure. (Bar = 5 μm)

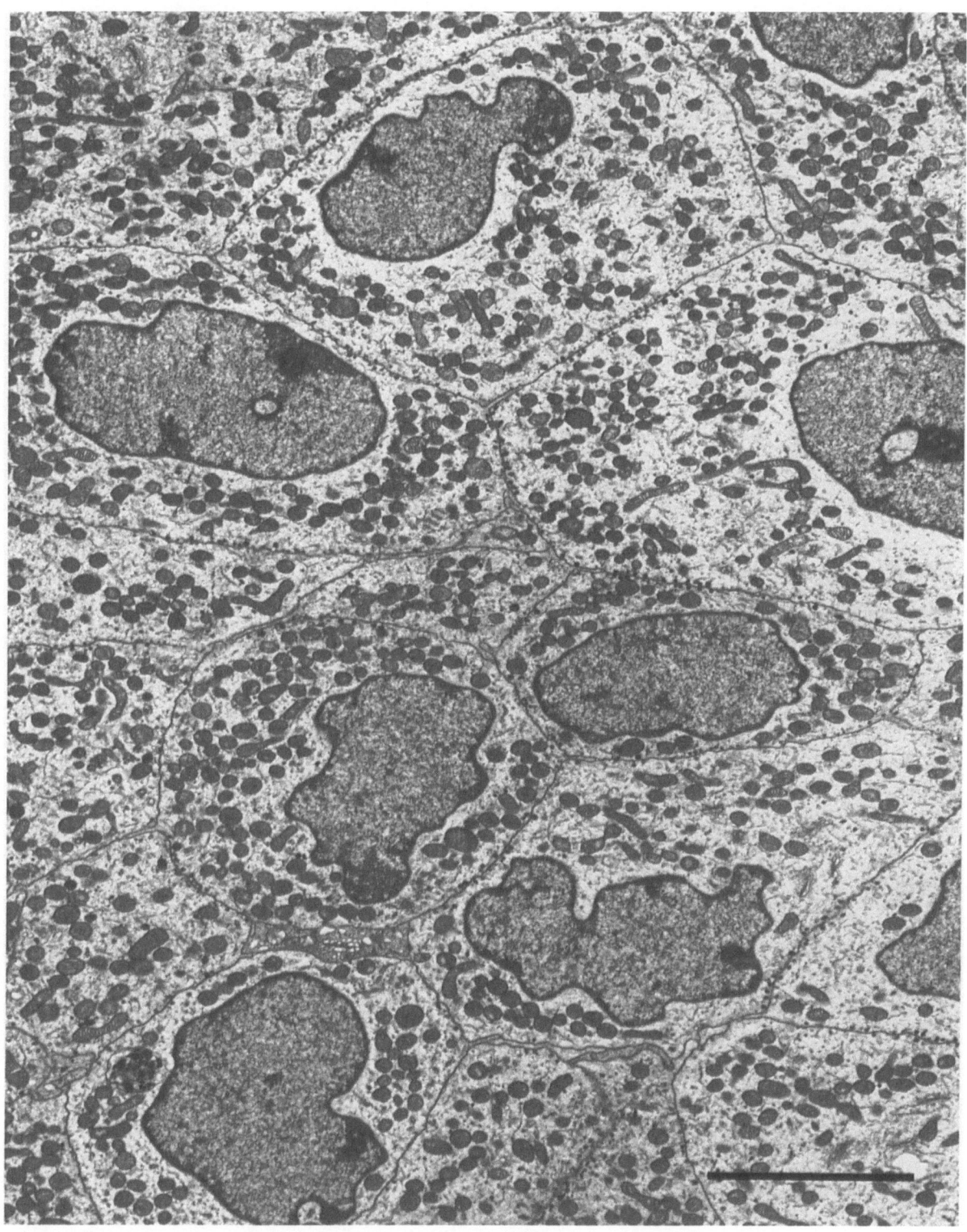

Fig. 21.8. *Pituitary adenoma.* Non-secretory tumour. The neurosecretory granules in these tumours are very sparse and small, usually measuring less than 100 nm across. In this figure they are visible only as tiny black dots lined up along the cell membranes. Other organelles are also normally scanty, but occasionally the cells show oncocytic change, as in this example, and contain abundant mitochondria. (Bar = 5 μm)

22 Primary Cerebral Lymphoma

Primary cerebral lymphomas have a similar ultra-structural appearance to systemic non-Hodgkin lymphomas, although they lack some of the architectural features of lymphomas arising within lymph nodes. The origin of the neoplastic lymphoid cells in these tumours and their relationship to central nervous system microglia is obscure. There is also no general agreement on the classification of these lymphomas at present, but most cases appear to consist of a mixed population of lymphoid cells, with variable predominance of smaller or larger cell types.

The smallest tumour cells present are ultra-structurally similar to poorly differentiated small lymphocytes. They have large, rounded nuclei with prominently clumped chromatin, and a scanty rim of perinuclear cytoplasm almost entirely filled by polyribosomes. There are no basement membranes or junctional attachments, but many examples show small, villous-like cytoplasmic projections. In most tumours there is also a spectrum of larger cell types, similar to the small lymphocytic cells but with irregularly indented or cleaved nuclei and more abundant perinuclear cytoplasm. These larger cells usually contain more numerous and varied organelles, including lysosomal vacuoles, and the cytoplasmic membrane may be prominently ruffled or deeply indented. The largest cells present may resemble phagocytes, and have very abundant, electron-dense cytoplasm packed with membrane-bound phagocytic processes which insinuate between the more lymphocytoid tumour cells. Plasma cells are also present in some cases, with eccentric nuclei and cytoplasm filled by parallel stacks of rough endoplasmic reticulum. Some lymphocytoid cells may contain Russell bodies, which are discrete arrays of dilated endoplasmic reticulum cisternae filled with fibrillary, electron-dense material.

In central areas the tumour cells are loosely arranged in sheets, but more peripherally small groups of infiltrating cells are often interspersed with astrocytic processes or more widely separated by pre-existing neuropil. These groups of infiltrating cells have a marked tendency to be centred on small blood vessels, and often form a discrete cuff of cells around the intact outer basement membrane of small capillaries. Larger blood vessels within these tumours typically have an expanded perivascular space which is filled by tumour cells lying inside the outer basement membrane. In either case, the tumour cells around blood vessels are often enclosed by patchily reduplicated vascular basement membrane. Together with the amorphous and fibrillary material present in the perivascular spaces, this reduplicated basement membrane represents the ultrastructural equivalent of the proliferated reticulin seen around cerebral lymphoma vessels on light microscopy.

Further Reading

Cervós-Navarro J, Matakas F (1975) The ultrastructure of reticulin. Acta Neuropathol [Suppl] VI: 173–176

Cravioto H (1975) Human and experimental reticulum cell sarcoma (microglioma) of the nervous system. Acta Neuropathol [Suppl] VI: 135–140

Hirano A, Ghatak NR, Becker NH, Zimmerman HM (1974) A comparison of the fine structure of small blood vessels in intracranial and retroperitoneal malignant lymphomas. Acta Neuropathol 27: 93–104

Ishida Y (1975) Fine structure of primary reticulum cell sarcoma of the brain. Acta Neuropathol [Suppl] VI: 147–153

Jellinger K, Slowick F, Sluga E (1979) Primary intracranial malignant lymphomas. A fine structural, cytochemical and CSF immunological study. Clin Neurol Neurosurg 81: 173–184

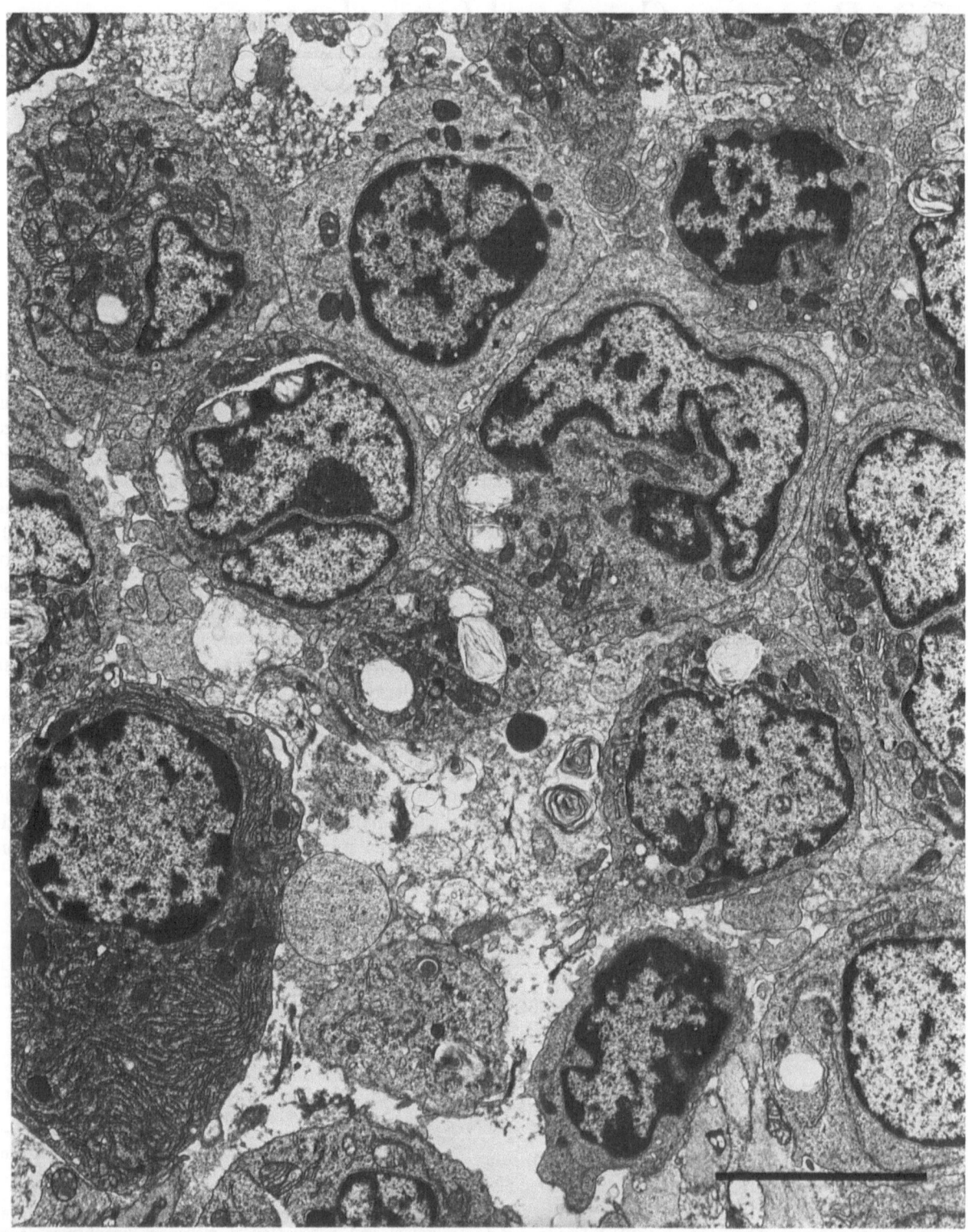

Fig. 22.1. *Primary cerebral lymphoma.* Most of these tumours consist of a mixed population of lymphocytoid cells loosely arranged in sheets, as in the example illustrated here. The smallest cells present resemble poorly differentiated small lymphocytes, with rounded nuclei and only a scanty rim of perinuclear cytoplasm. The larger cells have irregular or cleaved nuclei and more abundant cytoplasm containing increased organelles. Plasma cells are also occasionally present, and one can be seen at the *bottom left*. (Bar = 5 μm)

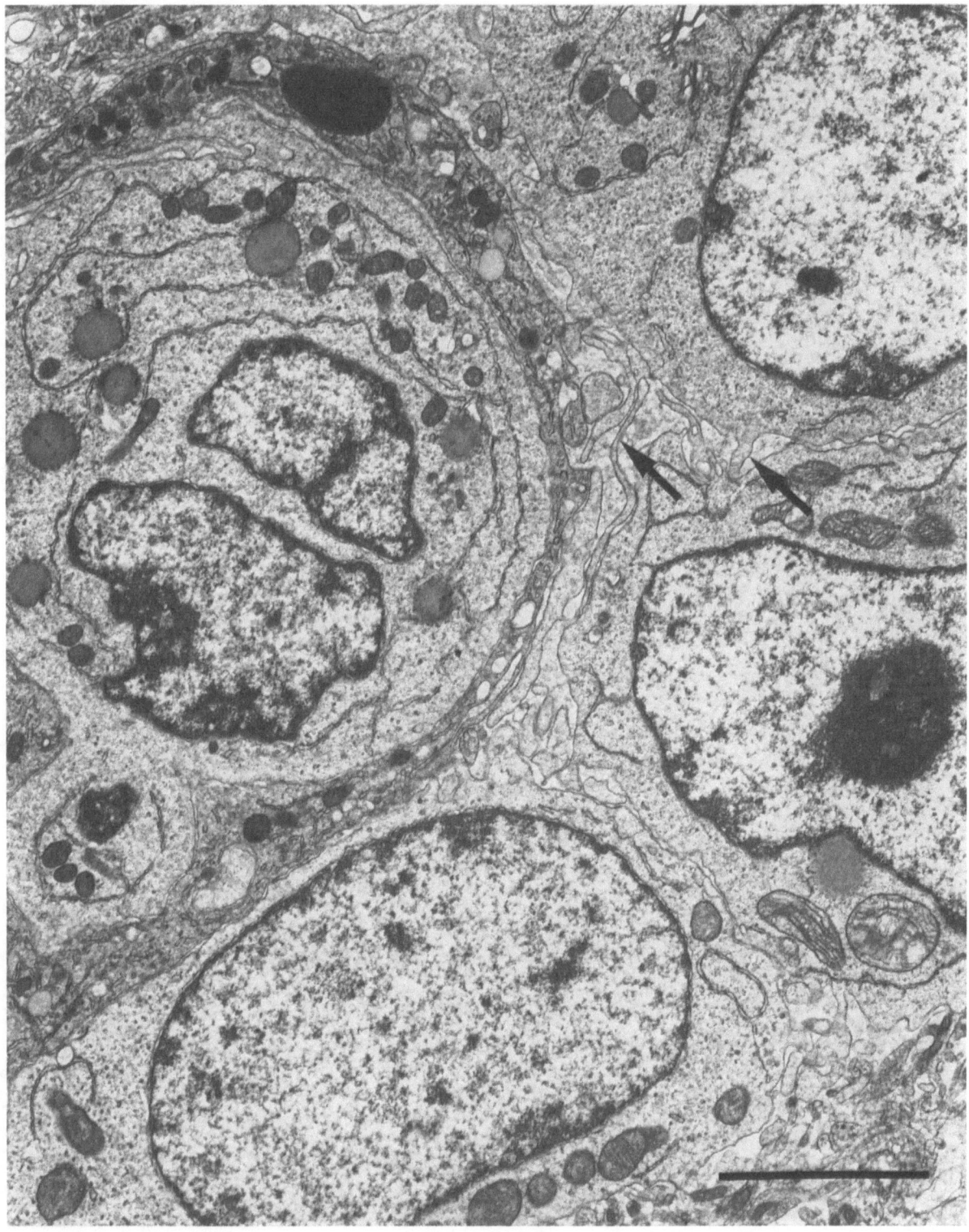

Fig. 22.2. *Primary cerebral lymphoma.* Tumour cells lack junctional attachments but may show peripheral villous projections, or irregular infoldings of the plasma membrane (*arrows*). Larger cells often have deeply cleaved nuclei, like the cell at the *top left*. This cell is enclosed by a typical, phagocytic-type cell process, with irregular, electron-dense cytoplasm containing abundant organelles. (Bar = 5 μm)

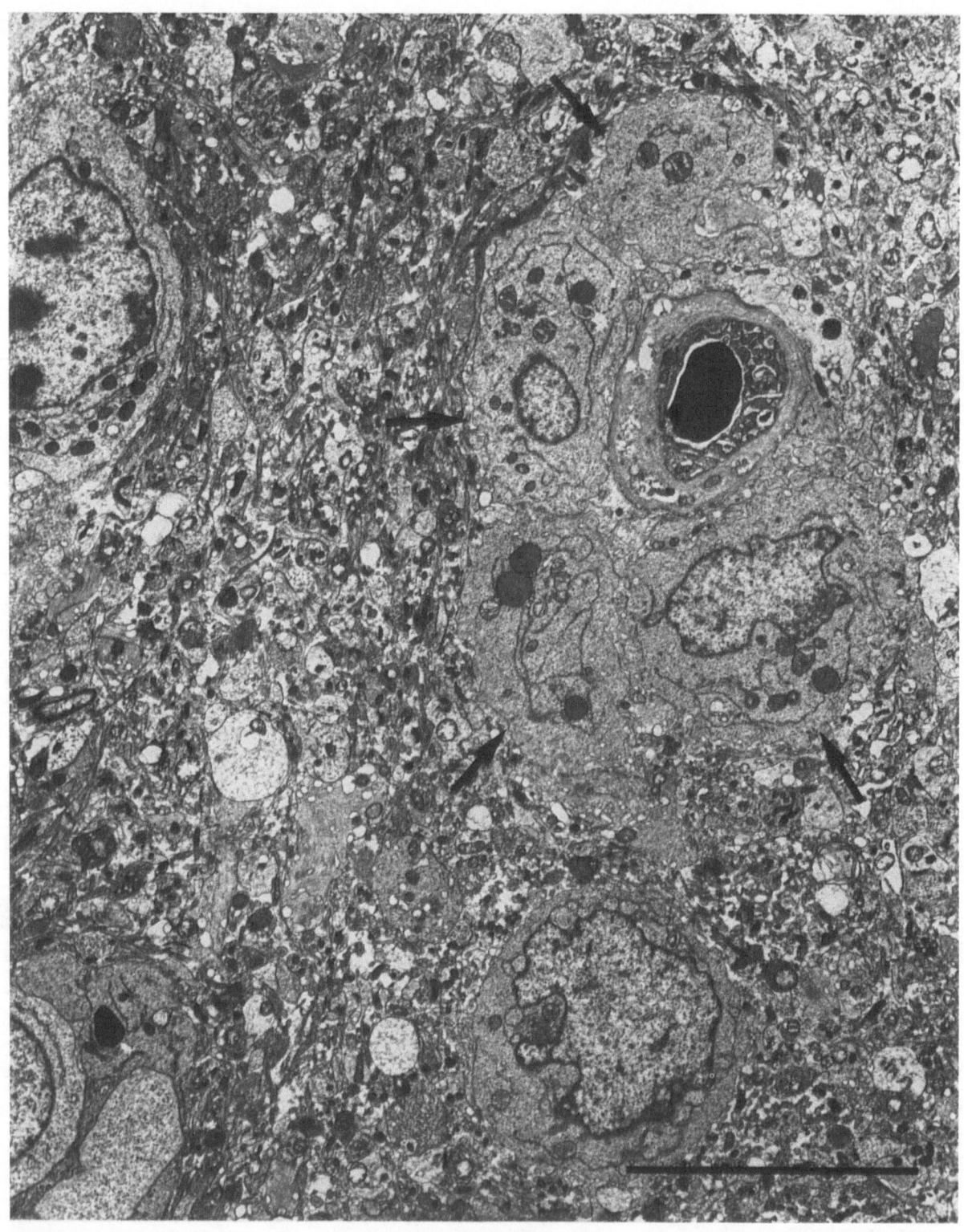

Fig. 22.3. *Primary cerebral lymphoma.* In diffusely infiltrated areas of brain, like that shown here, small groups of tumour cells are often widely separated by the pre-existing neuropil. These groups may be centred on capillary vessels, as at the *top right*, and often form a discrete cuff of tumour cells (*arrows*) which encloses the outer vascular basement membrane. (Bar = 10 μm)

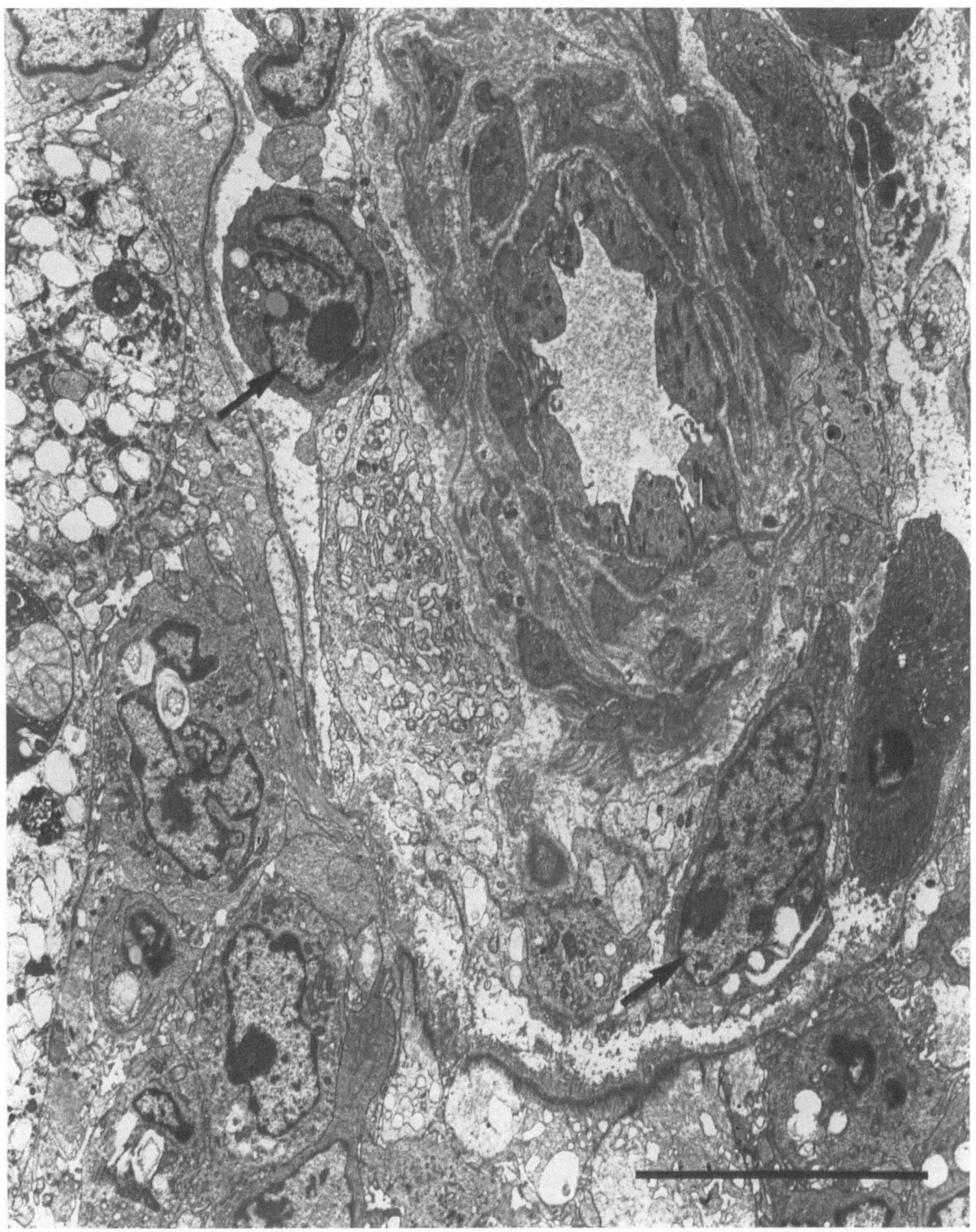

Fig. 22.4. *Primary cerebral lymphoma.* Larger blood vessels, like that in the *upper part* of this figure, often have an expanded perivascular space and tumour cells lying within the outer basement membrane (*arrows*). The perivascular space also contains amorphous and fibrillary material. Together with reduplicated basement membrane this material constitutes the ultrastructural equivalent of the proliferated reticulin seen on light microscopy. (Bar = 10 μm)

23 Secondary Carcinoma

Carcinomas are the most common type of secondary tumour found in the central nervous system, and although they may be the result of direct spread from a local primary site such as the mastoid antrum, they are most often distant metastases spread by a haematogenous route. In either case, the ultrastructural features of these secondary deposits are identical to those of carcinomas elsewhere in the body, and the appearances vary widely depending on the site of the primary tumour and the degree of of differentiation in the metastases. In most instances, however, a number of basic features can be identified at electron microscopic level which enable secondary carcinoma deposits to be distinguished from other central nervous system tumours, including choroid plexus carcinomas (see Chapter 8).

The tumour cells are typically arranged in mosaic or pavement-like sheets, and are linked by prominent, usually well-formed desmosomes. The perivascular and other extracellular spaces often contain collagen, which may be a prominent feature. Nuclei tend to be large and irregular, with finely granular chromatin and prominent nucleoli. The perinuclear cytoplasm is usually abundant, especially in the better differentiated examples, and patchy basement membrane surrounds the cells in some cases. Cytoplasmic organelles are extremely variable, but polyribosomes are often predominant and numerous enlarged mitochondria may also be a feature. In addition, most cells contain loose bundles of 5- to 10-nm intermediate filaments, sometimes referred to as tonofilaments or keratohyaline filaments.

Adenocarcinomas are more frequently encountered as central nervous system metastases than squamous carcinomas. Their cells usually contain fewer tonofilaments than those of squamous lesions, but there is typically more abundant rough endoplasmic reticulum and Golgi apparatus. The cells often form peripheral microvilli, and in well-differentiated tumour deposits they may be joined by apical desmosomes to form extracellular acini. Intracytoplasmic lumina lined by microvilli are also a characteristic ultrastructural feature of adenocarcinomas, although these may possibly simply represent deep membrane invaginations which have been cross-cut. Squamous carcinomas usually have larger numbers of desmosomes than adenocarcinomas, and intracytoplasmic tonofilaments are also typically more abundant. The filaments in squamous carcinomas often have a tendency to be aggregated into prominent, separate bundles, and in some cases these may form large, electron-dense bodies, or "keratohyaline granules".

Further Reading

Ghadially FN (1980) Diagnosis electron microscopy of tumours. Butterworths, London, pp 51–77
Trump BF, Jesudason ML, Jones RT (1978) Ultrastructural features of diseased cells: neoplasia. In: Trump BF, Jones RT (eds) Diagnostic electron microscopy, vol 1. John Wiley, New York, pp 54–64

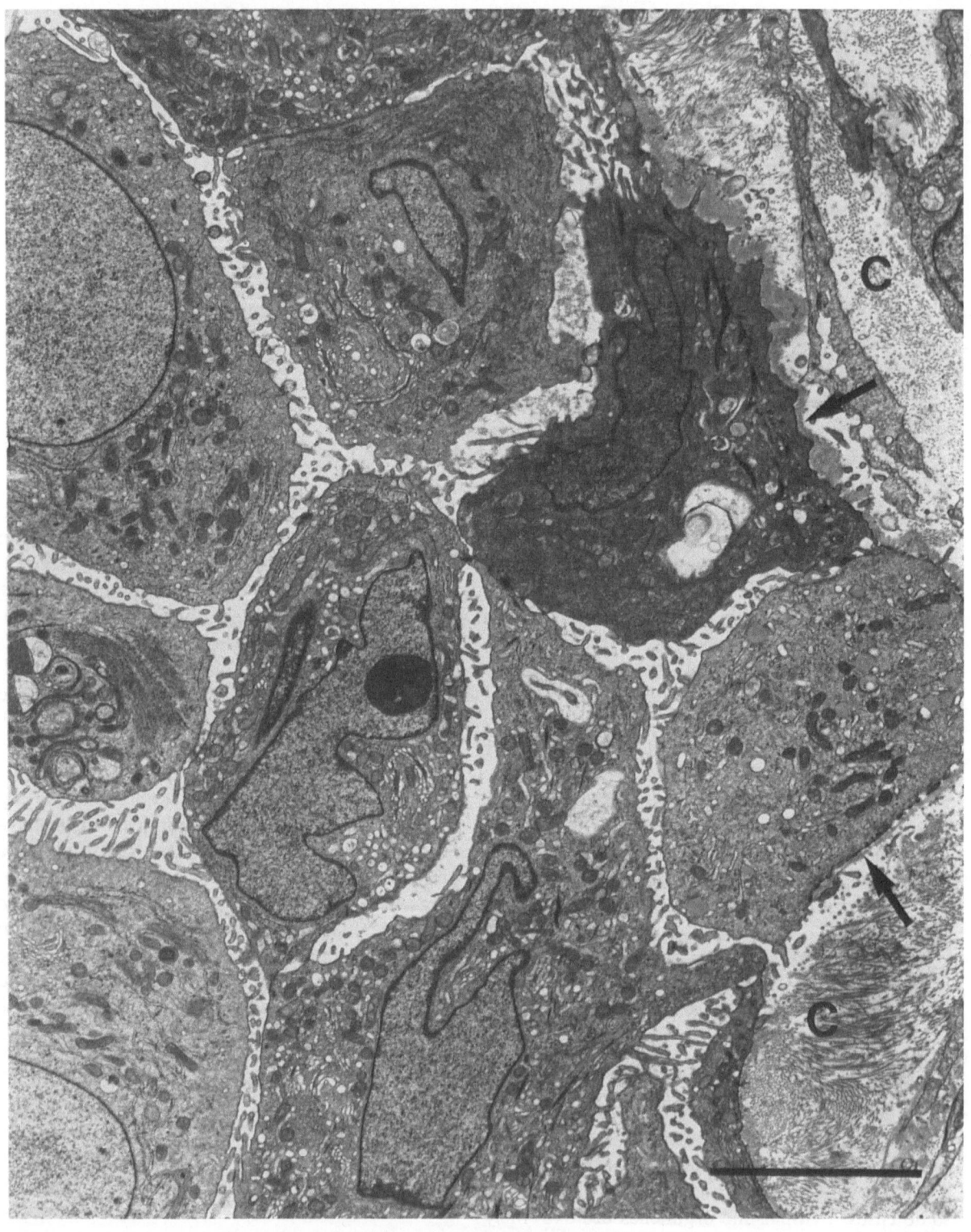

Fig. 23.1. *Secondary adenocarcinoma.* The cells are typically arranged in mosaic-like sheets and have abundant cytoplasm bearing numerous microvilli. As seen on the *far right*, there is usually abundant collagen (*C*) in the perivascular spaces, and tumour cells may be separated from this by patchy basement membrane (*arrows*). (Bar = 5 μm)

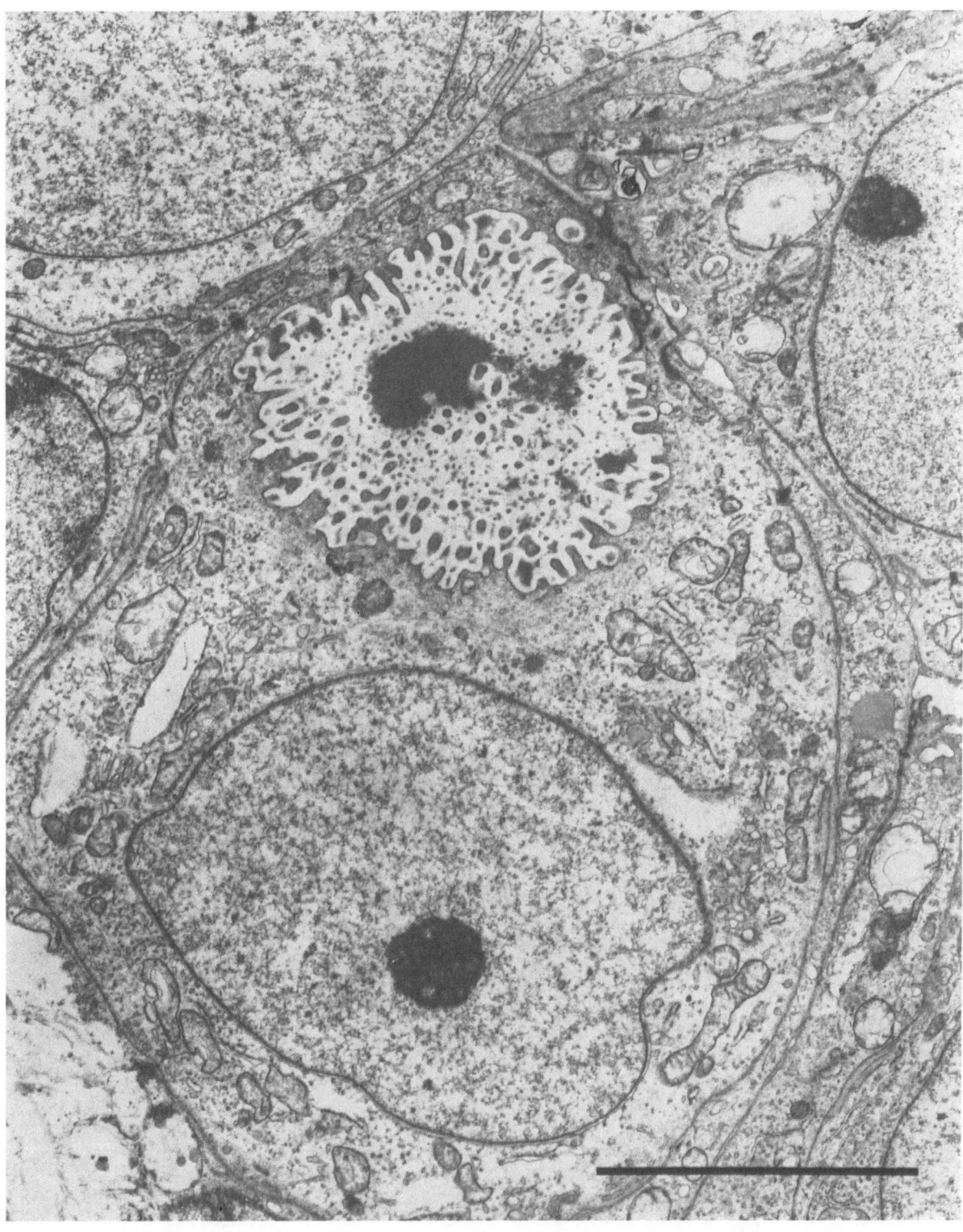

Fig. 23.2. *Secondary adenocarcinoma.* The cell nuclei are often large relative to the overall cell size, and typically have finely granular chromatin with prominent nucleoli. A characteristic feature of adenocarcinomas is the presence of intracytoplasmic lumina lined by microvilli, like that seen in the upper part of this figure. These lumina may be true intracytoplasmic structures, but it is also possible that they represent deep membrane invaginations which have been cross-cut. (Bar = 5 μm)

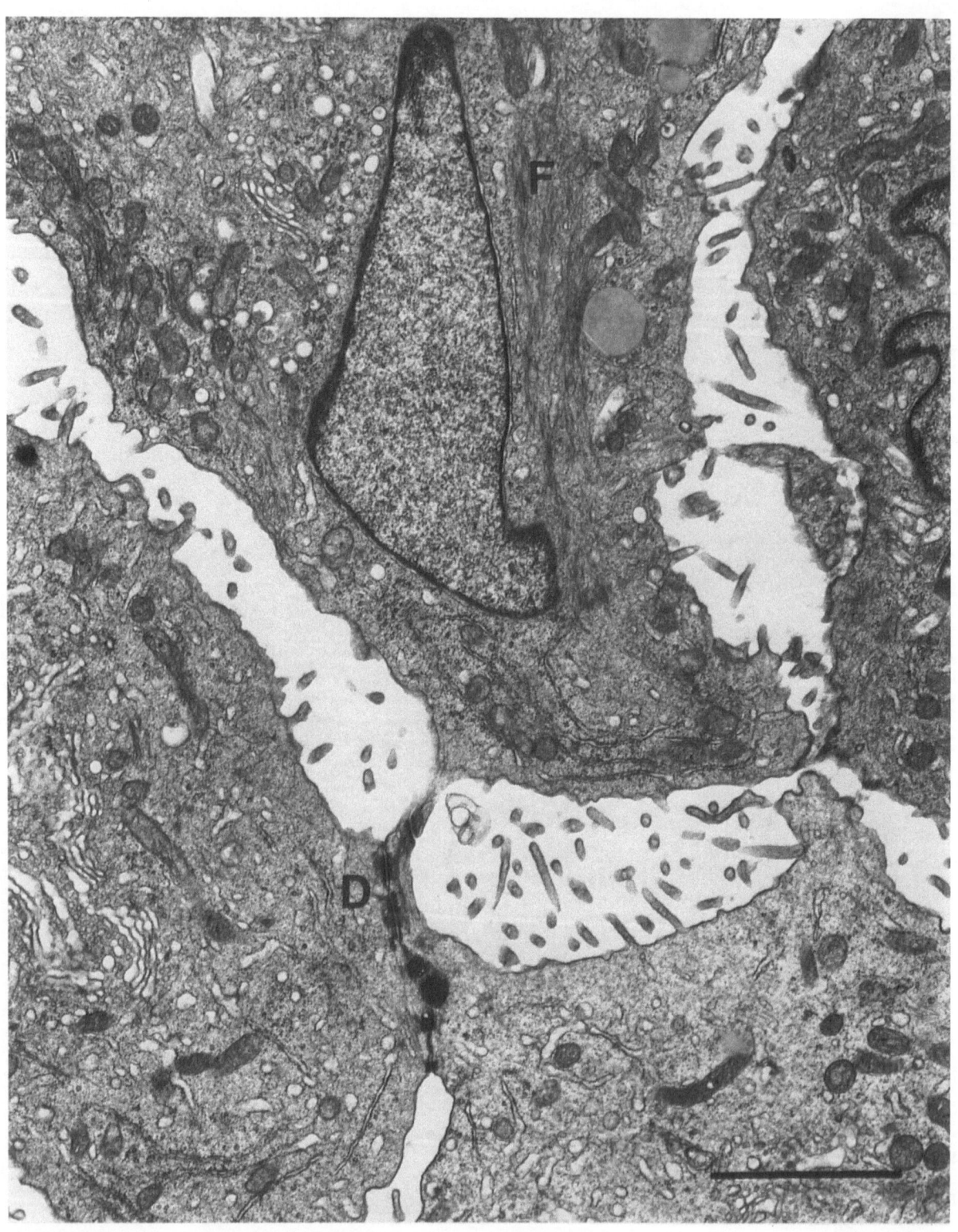

Fig. 23.3. *Secondary adenocarcinoma.* Adenocarcinoma cells often contain abundant Golgi apparatus, as in the cell on the *left.* In all types of carcinoma, the cells are usually joined by well-defined desmosomes (*D*) and also contain 5-nm tonofilaments, like those in the uppermost cell here (*F*). Both these features, however, are typically more prominent in squamous carcinomas. (Bar = 2 μm)

24 Sarcoma

Sarcomas of any type in the brain and spinal cord are most often secondary tumours resulting from local or metastatic spread, but in rare instances some examples may have a primary origin within the central nervous system. Such primary sarcomas may be primitive, polymorphic round-cell tumours, or more typical spindle-cell types, including leiomyosarcomas. Rhabdomyosarcomas may also occur as primary tumours, either taking origin within non-neoplastic leptomeninges or occurring within otherwise typical cerebellar medulloblastomas ("medullomyoblastomas"). Both the primary and the secondary sarcomas have ultrastructural appearances similar to those arising elsewhere in the body, and although there may be considerable variation between tumours of different soft tissue types, most spindle-cell sarcomas show some common distinguishing features at electron microscopic level.

The cell bodies can be very pleomorphic, but are often elongate, showing only a thin rim of cytoplasm when cut in cross-section. Nuclei are typically large, with an irregular outline. Cytoplasmic organelles are very variable, but pinocytotic vesicles are often a prominent feature and in many tumour types the cells also contain randomly arranged, thin cytoplasmic filaments, 6 to 8 nm in diameter. Basement membrane typically surrounds the cells, although it is patchy or absent in some types of tumour. Cells are usually separated by extracellular spaces containing abundant collagen, and in contrast to carcinomas, most types of spindle-cell sarcoma lack desmosomes or other junctional attachments.

In leiomyosarcomas, the nuclei often show a characteristic, concertina-like folding of the nuclear membrane, and both pinocytotic vesicles and 6- to 8-nm filaments are typically very abundant. In well-differentiated examples, multiple electron-dense foci may be scattered throughout the cytoplasm or lie adjacent to the inner aspect of the cell membranes. These are similar to the densities found in normal smooth muscle cells, and are formed by aggregation of focally thickened filaments.

Rhabdomyosarcomas tend to have larger, more pleomorphic cells than many other sarcomas and in sufficiently differentiated cases both thick (12–15 nm) and thin (6–8 nm) filaments are present together, often alternating with each other. Free ribosomes have a characteristic tendency to line up along the filaments in "Indian file", and electron-dense foci resembling Z-band material may occasionally be associated with individual bundles of filaments. In very well-differentiated tumours, this electron-dense material may form periodic transverse bars across long bundles of thick and thin filaments, producing structures which resemble primitive sarcomeres.

Further Reading

Ferenczy A, Rickart RM (1979) Leiomyoma and leiomyosarcoma. In: Trump BJ, Jones RT (eds) Diagnostic electron microscopy, vol 2. John Wiley, New York, pp 285–289

Ghadially FN (1980) Diagnostic electron microscopy of tumours. Butterworths, London, pp 128–130

Hinton DR, Halliday WC (1984) Primary rhabdomyosarcoma of the cerebellum. A light, electron microscopic and immunohistochemical study. J Neuropathol Exp Neurol 43: 439–449

Morales AR, Fine G, Horn RC Jr (1972) Rhabdomyosarcoma: an ultrastructural re-appraisal. Pathol Annu 7: 81–106

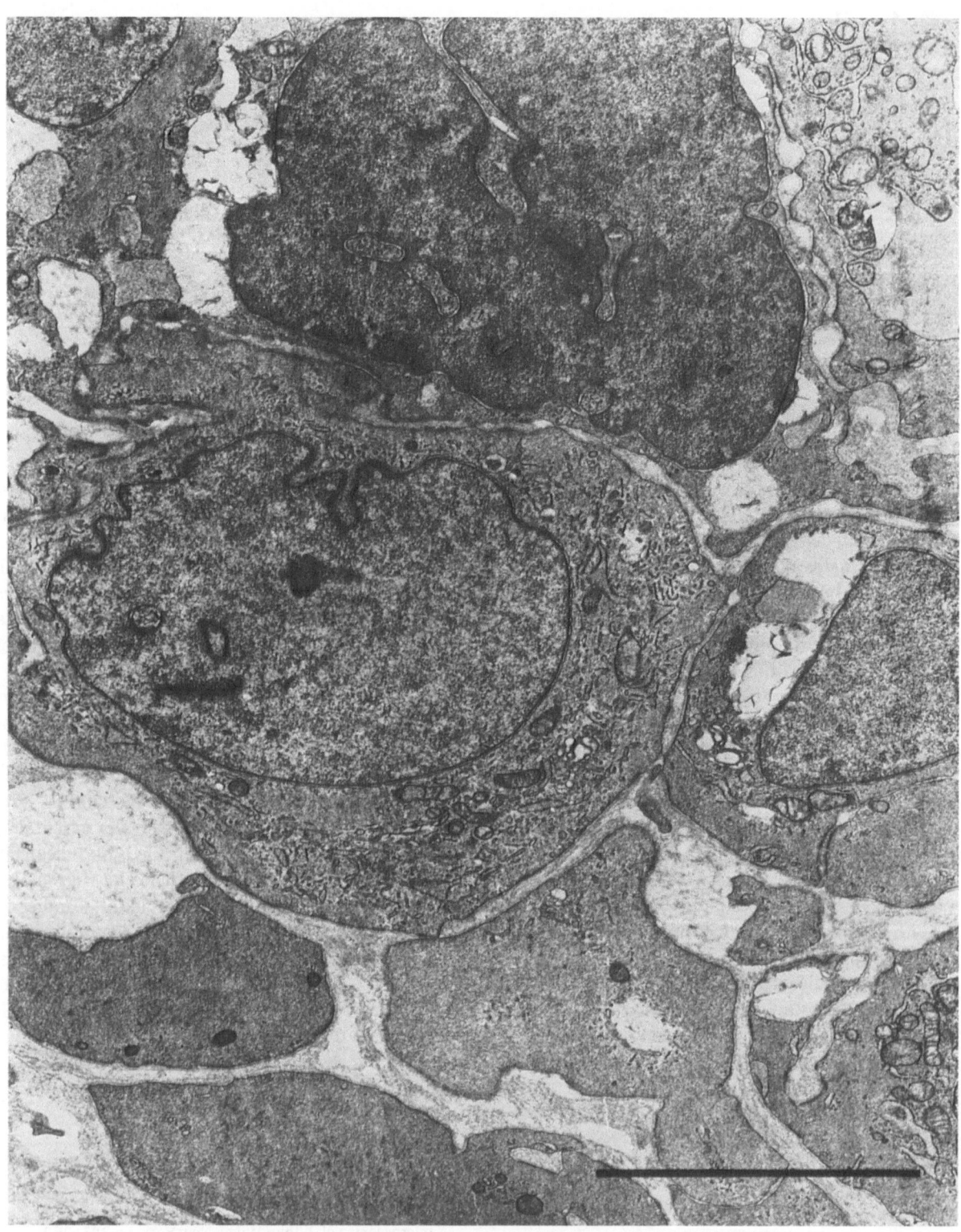

Fig. 24.1. *Leiomyosarcoma*. The cells are typically elongate and spindle shaped, but when seen in cross-section like this they appear rounded, with only a thin rim of perinuclear cytoplasm. Nuclei are usually large and often show a characteristic concertina-like folding of the nuclear membrane, similar to that seen in the central cell here. As in many spindle-cell sarcomas, there are no membrane junctions and the cells are separated by extracellular space containing abundant collagen. This figure and Fig. 24.2 are from a primary leiomyosarcoma arising within the cerebellum. (Bar = 5 μm)

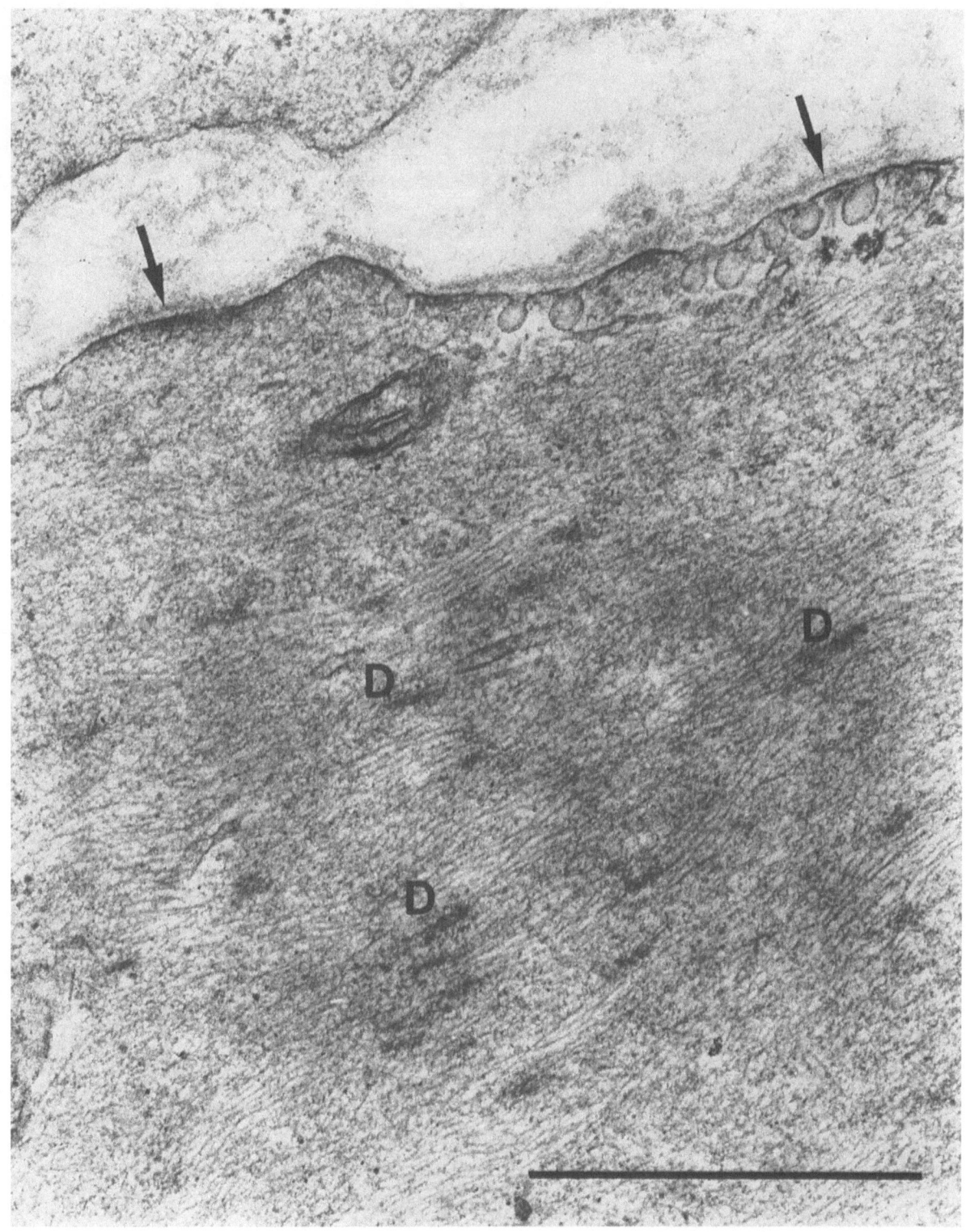

Fig. 24.2. *Leiomyosarcoma.* Tumour cells are usually surrounded by an intact basement membrane (*arrows*), and beneath this there are often abundant pinocytotic vesicles in the cytoplasm, visible along the upper margin of this cell. Thin, 6- to 8-nm cytoplasmic filaments may be found in many sarcomas but are often particularly abundant in leiomyosarcomas, and may aggregate to form multiple focal densities (*D*) in well-differentiated cells. (Bar = 1 μm)

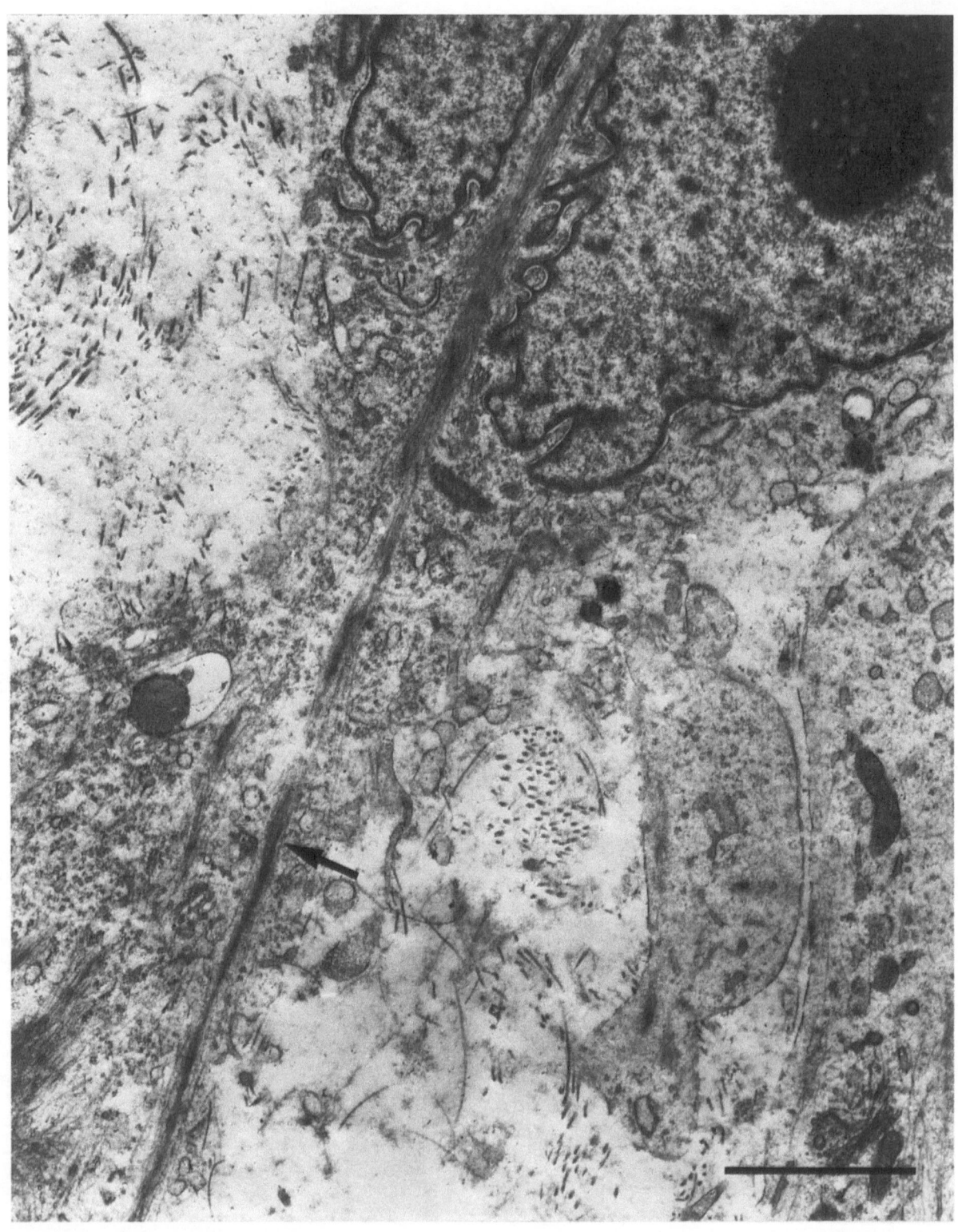

Fig. 24.3. *Rhabdomyosarcoma*. The cells tend to be more pleomorphic than in many other sarcomas and may have lobulated nuclei, as in this example. In elongated "strap-cells" like the one shown here, cytoplasmic filaments may be aligned in narrow bundles running down the long axis of the cell (*arrow*). This figure and Figs. 24.4 and 24.5 are from an intracranial tumour originating from an orbital muscle. (Bar = 2 μm)

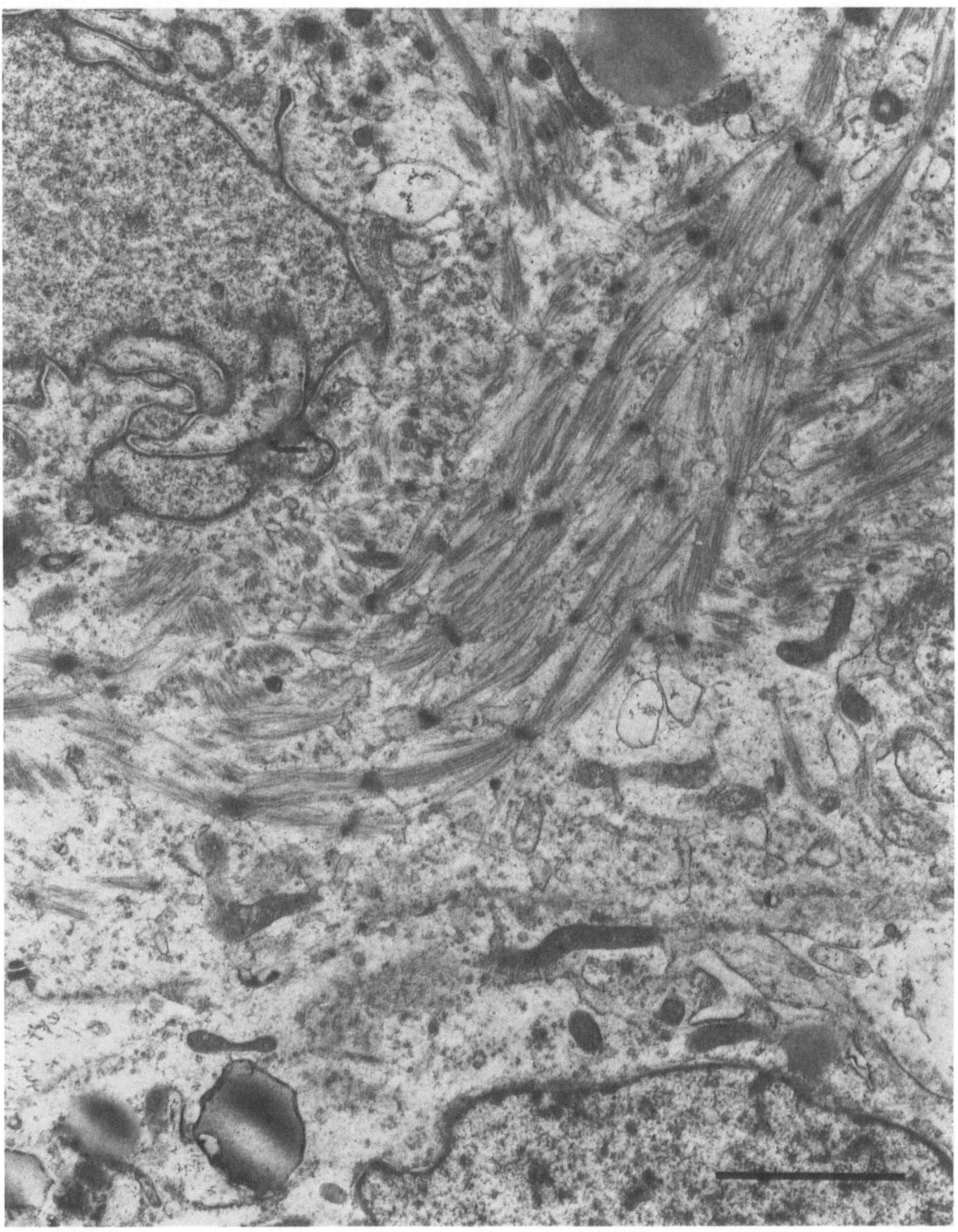

Fig. 24.4. *Rhabdomyosarcoma.* Separate, randomly orientated bundles of filaments are sometimes associated with discrete, electron-dense foci resembling Z-band material, visible as dark spots in this cell. The appearances are reminiscent of disorientated, primitive sarcomeres. (Bar = 2 μm)

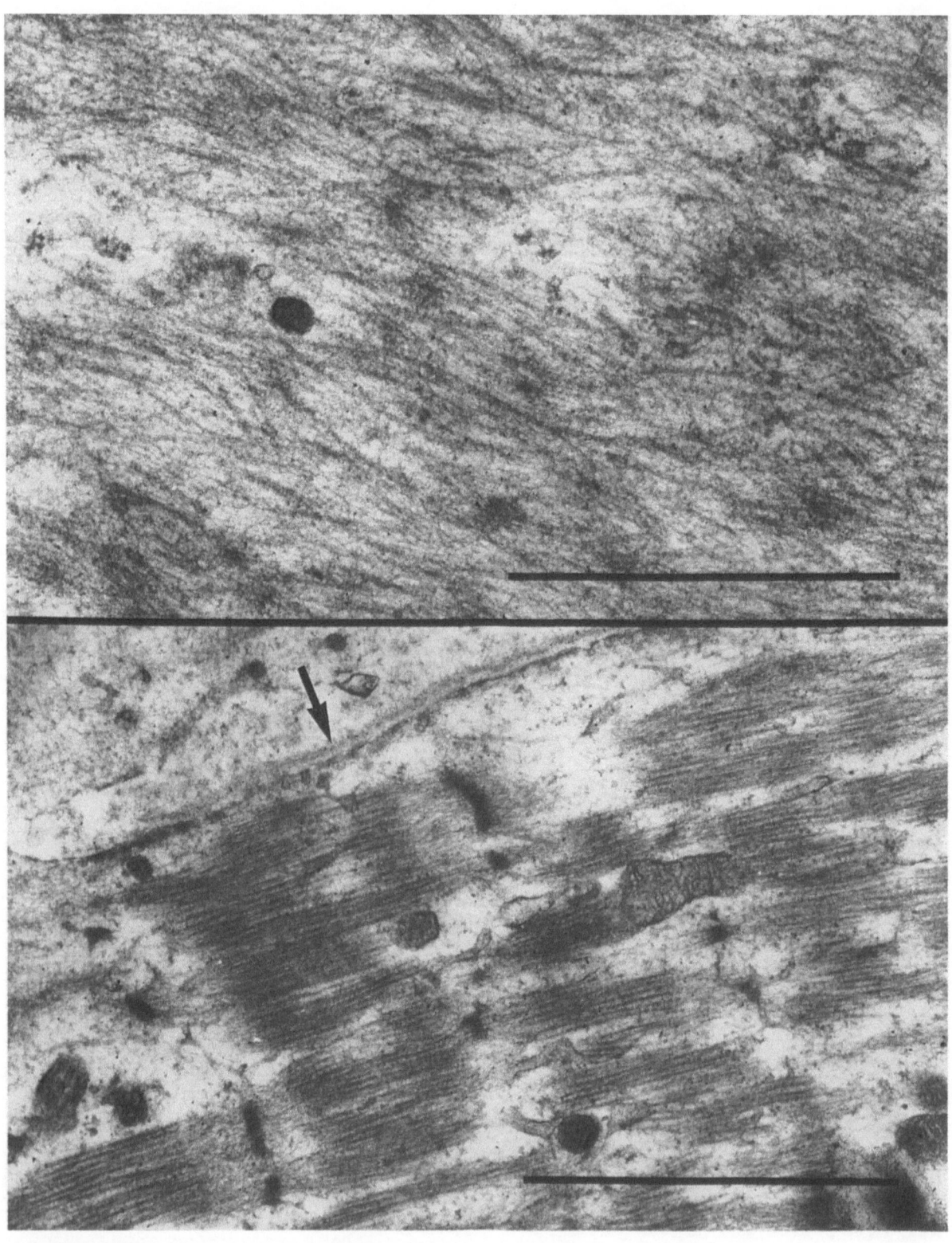

Fig. 24.5. *Rhabdomyosarcoma. Top*: Both thick (12–15 nm) and thin (6–8 nm) filaments may occur together in well-differentiated cells, and both are needed to make a definite diagnosis of rhabdomyosarcoma. (Bar = 1 μm) *Bottom*: In very well-differentiated tumours, electron-dense material may form periodic transverse bars across bundles of alternating thick and thin filaments, producing distinct sarcomere-like structures like these. Such tumour cells usually have an intact basement membrane (*arrow*). (Bar = 2 μm)

Bibliography

Azzarelli B, Rekate HL, Roessmann U (1977) Subependymoma. A case report with ultrastructural study. Acta Neuropathol 40: 279–282

Azzarelli B, Richards O, Anton AH, Roessmann U (1977) Central neuroblastoma. Electron microscopic observations and catecholamine determinations. J Neuropathol Exp Neurol 36: 384–397

Boesel CP, Suhan JP (1979) A pigmented choroid plexus carcinoma: histochemical and ultrastructural studies. J Neuropathol Exp Neurol 38: 177–186

Carter LP, Beggs J, Waggener JD (1972) Ultrastructure of three choroid plexus papillomas. Cancer 30: 1130–1136

Castaigne P, David M, Petuiset B, Escourolle R, Poirier J (1968) L'Ultrastructure des hémangioblastomes du système nerveux central. Rev Neurol 118: 5–26

Cervós-Navarro J (1971) Elektronenmikroskopie der Hämangioblastome des ZNS und der angioblastische Meningiome. Acta Neuropathol 19: 184–207

Cervós-Navarro J (1981) Ultrastructure of oligodendrogliomas. Acta Neuropathol [Suppl] 7: 91–93

Cervós-Navarro J, Matakas F (1975) The ultrastructure of reticulin. Acta Neuropathol [Suppl] VI: 173–176

Cervós-Navarro J, Vasquez JJ (1969) An electron microscopic study of meningiomas. Acta Neuropathol 13: 301–323

Cravioto H (1969) The ultrastructure of acoustic nerve tumours. Acta Neuropathol 12: 116–140

Cravioto H (1975) Human and experimental reticulum cell sarcoma (microglioma) of the nervous system. Acta Neuropathol [Suppl] VI: 135–140

Cravioto H, Dart D (1973) The ultrastructure of "pinealomas" (seminoma-like tumour of the pineal region), J Neuropathol Exp Neurol 32: 552–565

Cummins MB, Cravioto HM, Epstein F, Ransohoff J (1980) Medulloblastoma: an ultrastructural study—evidence for astrocytic and neuronal differentiation. Neurosurg 6: 398–411

DeCicco A, Dekker A, Yunis EJ (1972) Fine structure of Crooke's hyaline change in the human pituitary gland. Arch Pathol 94: 65–70

Dohrman GJ, Bucy PC (1970) Human choroid plexus: a light and electron microscopic study. J Neurosurg 33: 506–516

Dolman CL (1984) Ultrastructure of brain tumours and biopsies. Praeger, New York, pp 85–105

Doniach I (1972) Cytology of pituitary adenomas. JR Coll Phys Lond 6: 299–308

Duffell D, Farber L, Chou S, Hartmann JF, Nelson F (1963) Electron microscopic observations on astrocytomas. Subependymal glomerulate astrocytoma. Am J Pathol 43: 539–545

Ebhardt G, Cervós-Navarro J (1981) The fine structure of cells in astrocytomas of various grades of malignancy. Acta Neuropathol 7: 88–90

Erlandson RA, Woodruff JM (1982) Peripheral nerve sheath tumours: an electron microscopic study of 43 cases. Cancer 49: 273–287

Erlandson RA, Tandler B, Lieberman PM, Higinbotham NO (1968) Ultrastructure of human chordoma. Cancer Res 28: 2115–2125

Esiri MM, Adams CBT, Burke C, Underdown R (1983) Pituitary adenomas: immunohistology and ultrastructural analysis of 118 tumours. Acta Neuropathol 62: 1–14

Ferenczy A, Rickart RM (1979) Leiomyoma and leiomyosarcoma. In: Trump BJ, Jones RT (eds) Diagnostic electron microscopy, vol 2. Wiley, New York, pp 285–289

Fu YS, Chen ATL, Kay S, Young HF (1974) Is subependymoma (subependymal glomerulate astrocytoma) an astrocytoma or an ependymoma? A comparative ultrastructural and tissue culture study. Cancer 34: 1992–2008

Garcia JH, Lemini H (1970) Ultrastructure of oligodendroglioma of the spinal cord. Am J Clin Pathol 54: 757–765

Ghadially FN (1980) Diagnostic electron microscopy of tumours. Butterworths, London

Ghatak NR, Hirano A, Zimmerman HM (1971) Ultrastructure of a craniopharyngioma. Cancer 27: 1465–1475

Goebel HH, Cravioto H (1972) Ultrastructure of human and experimental ependymomas. J Neuropathol Exp Neurol 31: 55–71

Gonatus NK, Besen M (1963) An electron microscopic study of three human psammomatous meningiomas. J Neuropathol Exp Neurol 22: 263–273

Grisoli F, Vincentelli F, Boudouresques G, Delpuech F, Hassoun J, Raybaud C (1981) Primary cerebral neuroblastoma in an adult man. Surg Neurol 16: 266–270

Gullotta F, DeMelo AS (1979) Carcinomas and malignant papillomas of the choroid plexus. Neurochir (Stuttg) 22: 1–9

Hassoun J, Gambarelli D, Peragut JC, Toga M (1983) Specific

ultrastructural markers of human pinealomas. Acta Neuropathol 62: 31–40

Herrick MK, Rubinstein LJ (1979) The cytological differentiating potential of pineal parenchymal neoplasms (true pinealomas). A clinicopathological study of 28 tumours. Brain 102: 289–320

Hess JR (1978) Frequency of surface microprojections and coated vesicles with increased malignancy in human astrocytic neoplasms. Acta Neuropathol 44: 151–153

Hinton DR, Halliday WC (1984) Primary rhabdomyosarcoma of the cerebellum. A light, electron microscopic and immunohistochemical study. J Neuropathol Exp Neurol 43: 439–449

Hirano A, Ghatak NR, Wisoff HS, Zimmerman HM (1971) Comparative ultrastructural study of ependymoma and ependymal cyst. Am J Pathol 62: 11a

Hirano A, Ghatak NR, Becker NH, Zimmerman HM (1974) A comparison of the fine structure of small blood vessels in intracranial and retroperitoneal malignant lymphomas. Acta Neuropathol 27: 93–104

Ho K-L (1985) Eccordosis physaliphora and chordoma: A comparative ultrastructural study. Clin Neuropathol 4: 77–86

Hossmann KA, Wechsler W (1971) Ultrastructural cytopathology of human cerebral gliomas. Oncology 25: 455–480

Ishida Y (1975) Fine structure of primary reticulum cell sarcoma of the brain. Acta Neuropathol [Suppl] VI: 147–153

Jellinger K (1978) Glioblastoma multiforme: morphology and biology. Acta Neurochir (Wein) 42: 5–32

Jellinger J, Slowick F, Sluga E (1979) Primary intracranial malignant lymphomas. A fine structural, cytochemical and CSF immunological study. Clin Neurol Neurosurg 81: 173–184

Kawamura J, Garcia JH, Kamijo Y (1973) Cerebellar haemangioblastoma: histogenesis of stromal cells. Cancer 31: 1528–1540

Kepes J (1961) Electron microscopic studies of meningiomas. Am J Pathol 39: 499–510

Kline KT, Damjanor I, Katz SM, Schmidek H (1979) Pineoblastomas: an electron microscopic study. Cancer 44: 1692–1699

Landolt AM (1975) Ultrastructure of human sella tumours. Correlations of clinical findings and morphology. Acta Neurochir [Suppl] 22: 1–167

Lassmann H, Jurecka W, Lassmann G, Gebhart W, Matrash H, Watzek G (1977) Different types of benign nerve sheath tumours. Light microscopy, electron microscopy and autoradiography. Virchows Arch [A] 375: 197–210

Lee JC, Glasauer FE (1968) Ganglioglioma: light and electron microscopic study. Neurochir (Stuttg) 11: 160–170

Liu HM, McLone DG, Clark S (1977) Ependymomas of childhood. Childs Brain 3: 281–296

Luse SA (1960) Electron microscopic studies of brain tumours. Neurology 10: 881–905

Markesberry WR, Haugh RM, Young AB (1981) Ultrastructure of pineal parenchymal neoplasms. Acta Neuropathol 55: 143–149

Matakas F, Cervós-Navarro J, Gullota F (1976) The ultrastructure of medulloblastoma. Acta Neuropathol 16: 271–284

Morales AR, Fine G, Horn RC Jr (1972) Rhabdomyosarcoma: an ultrastructural re-appraisal. Pathol Annu 7: 81–106

Moss TH (1983) Electron microscopic observations on malignant choroid plexus papilloma. Neuropathol Appl Neurobiol 9: 225–235

Moss TH (1983) Evidence for differentiation in medulloblastomas appearing primitive on light microscopy: an ultrastructural study. Histopathology 7: 919–930

Moss TH (1984) Observations on the nature of subependymoma. An electron microscopic study. Neuropathol Appl Neurobiol 10: 63–75

Nakashima N, Goto J, Takeuchi J (1982) Papillary carcinomas of choroid plexus. Light and electron microscopic study. Virchows Arch [A] 395: 303–318

Napolitano L, Kyle R, Fisher ER (1963) Ultrastructure of meningiomas and the derivation and nature of their cellular components. Cancer 17: 233–241

Nielson SL, Wilson BB (1975) Ultrastructure of a 'pineocytoma'. J Neuropathol Exp Neurol 34: 148–158

Pĕna CE (1975) Intracranial haemangiopericytoma. Ultrastructural evidence of its leiomyoblastic differentiation. Acta Neuropathol 33: 279–284

Poirier J, Escourolle R, Castaigne P (1968) Les neurofibromas de la malodie de Recklinghausen. Étude ultrastructurale et place neurologique par rapport aux neurinomes. Acta Neuropathol 10: 279–294

Popoff NA, Malinn TI, Rosomoff ML (1974) Fine structure of intracranial haemangiopericytoma and angiomatous meningioma. Cancer 34: 1187–1197

Raimondi AJ, Mullan S, Evans JP (1962) Human brain tumours. An electron microscopic study. J Neurosurg 19: 731–753

Ramsey HJ (1965) Ultrastructure of pineal tumour. Cancer 18: 1014–1025

Rawlinson DG, Herman MM, Rubinstein LJ (1973) The fine structure of a myxopapillary ependymoma of the filum terminale. Acta Neuropathol 25: 1–13

Rhodes RH, Davis RL, Kassel SH, Clague BH (1978) Primary cerebral neuroblastoma: a light and electron microscopic study. Acta Neuropathol 41: 119–124

Robertson DM, Vogel FS (1962) Concentric lamination of glial processes in oligodendrogliomas. J Cell Biol 15: 313–334

Robertson DM, Hendry WS, Vogel FS (1964) Central ganglioneuroma: a case study using electron microscopy. J Neuropathol Exp Neurol 23: 692–705

Roy S (1977) An ultrastructural study of medulloblastoma. Neurol India 25: 226–229

Rubinstein LJ, Herman MM (1972) A light and electron microscopic study of a temporal lobe ganglioglioma. J Neurol Sci 16: 27–28

Rubinstein LJ, Herman MM, Hanberry JW (1974) The relationship between differentiating medulloblastoma and dedifferentiating diffuse cerebellar astrocytoma. Cancer 33: 675–690

Schober R, Nelson D (1975) Fine structure and origin of amyloid deposits in pituitary adenoma. Arch Pathol 99: 403–410

Shin WY, Laufer H, Lee YC, Aftalion B, Hirano A, Zimmermann HM (1978) Fine structure of a cerebellar neuroblastoma. Acta Neuropathol 42: 11–13

Sian CS, Ryan SF (1981) The ultrastructure of neurilemoma with emphasis on Antoni B tissue. Hum Pathol 12: 145–160

Spence AM, Rubinstein LJ (1975) Cerebellar capillary haemangioblastoma: its histogenesis studied by organ culture and electron microscopy. Cancer 35: 326–341

Tabuchi K, Yamada O, Nishimoto A (1973) The ultrastructure of pinealomas. Acta Neuropathol 24: 117–127

Tani E, Higashi N (1972) Intercellular junctions in human ependymomas. Acta Neuropathol 22: 295–304

Trump BF, Jesudason ML, Jones RT (1978) Ultrastructural features of diseased cells: neoplasia. In: Trump BF, Jones RT (eds) Diagnostic electron microscopy, vol 1. John Wiley, New York, pp 54–64

Waggener JD (1966) Ultrastructure of benign peripheral nerve sheath tumours. Cancer 19: 699–709

Wischnitzer S (1970) The annulate lamellus. Int Rev Cytol 27: 65–100

Wolfson WL, Brown WJ (1977) Disseminated choroid plexus papilloma. An ultrastructural study. Arch Pathol Lab Med 101: 366–368

Yagishita S, Itoh Y, Chiba, Yamishita T, Nakazima F, Kuwabara T (1980) Cerebellar neuroblastoma. A light and ultrastructural study. Acta Neuropathol 50: 139–142

Zülch KJ, Wechsler W (1968) Pathology and classification of gliomas. In: Kragenbuhl H, Maspes PE, Sweet WH (eds) Neurological surgery, vol 2. Karger, Basel, pp 1–84

Subject Index